ADVANCE PRAISE

"After all the years that I played in the MLB, I'm no stranger to great coaching—and the nutrition team at re:vitalize is among the best when it comes to nutrition and weight loss."

—MIGUEL MONTERO, two-time MLB
All-Star, World Series champion

"As a former professional cheerleader and now mom of three, I've tried all the diets and tricks of the trade, and nothing has ever worked except re:vitalize! Dr. Abood's approach was easy, straightforward, and the perfect roadmap to get back to the happy, healthier me!"

—JENNI CROFT, *Bachelor* season 11 finalist, Dallas Cowboy
cheerleader, Miami Heat dancer, mom of three

"This book will do for you what Dr. Abood and Dan have done for so many of my patients who have been wrestling with diabetes, high blood pressure, and other obesity-related diseases: take your nutrition and health to the next level. They will show you how to not only get back to your healthiest weight and self but enjoy food while doing it. I have unbelievable trust and faith in them both—and so should you."

—DR. TOM FIEL, former team physician for
the Phoenix Suns and Milwaukee Brewers

"In an industry that profits from failure, Noel and Dan at re:vitalize are invested in long-term health and wellness for their clients. Their integrity is so refreshing! Even when their clients want to keep losing, they encourage them to stop and let their bodies take a break. Trust them; they know what they are doing."

—DR. KARI ANDERSON, myeatingdoctor.com,
author of *food, body & love*

"Being on the road with a professional basketball team can make it challenging to keep unwanted weight off and difficult to decide on the 'right' foods to eat! Dr. Noel Abood, Dan LeMoine, and their team helped show me how to get the results I wanted in a short period of time and how to continue long after reaching my goals and to this very day. Check out this book if you find yourself needing to do the same!"

—AARON NELSON, VP of Player Care and
Performance, New Orleans Pelicans

"Since my playing days have been over, I've spent a lot of time in front of the camera and being a role model to other guys in the NBA. Dan and Noel have given me a blueprint to easily maintain my healthiest weight and keep myself in optimal shape. I'm as fit as I was when I was playing!"

—EDDIE JOHNSON, NBA great,
cohost of *NBA Today*

"The link between nutrition and performance is undeniable. Whether you're looking to perform on the field, in your career, or in life, nutrition is key. Dr. Abood and Dan taught me that customized nutrition is the fastest way to achieve your health and weight loss goals. I look great and feel so much younger after re:vitalize. It is a definite game-changer."

—DR. JOHN BADOLATO, *Extreme Makeover:
Weight Loss Edition*, team dentist for the Phoenix Suns
and Arizona Diamondbacks

"Most nutrition and weight loss programs are some combination of 'eat less and exercise more.' It's time we rethink how we approach effective, sustainable weight loss. Look no further than this book."

—DR. JOE DEKA, MD

"This book is a must-read if you care about your health and want to change your life! I am a former pro athlete who struggled with weight issues, up and down! Dan and Noel showed me how to lose the weight once and for all: forty-one pounds in forty days, and I kept it off."

—TIM KEMPTON, sportscaster, NBA great

"Covering professional sports and athletes day in and day out, the link between nutrition and performance is undeniable. Whether you're looking to perform on the field or in life, nutrition is key. This approach taught me that customized nutrition is the fastest way to achieve your health and weight loss goals."

—DAN BICKLEY, sports columnist, on-air radio host of the *Bickley & Marotta* show

"The re:vitalize team has found the right combination of emotional and mental support to layer over a sustainable health program that reshapes mind and body back to our true nature."

—DR. GREG SPEARS, DO

"I used to eat like a fourteen-year-old kid whose parents were out of town, so needless to say, I got heavy. I had doubts about whether or not I had the ability or discipline to lose weight, but the methods of Dr. Abood and his staff alleviated those doubts quickly—and changed my life in the process!"

—VINCE MAROTTA, cohost of *Bickley & Marotta*, ArizonaSports.com

"Eating healthy doesn't mean you can't enjoy delicious food. Doc and Dan's philosophy on whole-food nutrition will help you get healthy and still enjoy the food you love."

—CHEF MIKE DEI MAGGI, Executive Chef of the Phoenix Suns

Disclaimer:

Weight loss plans and programs can be transformational. The benefits—medically, psychologically, and physically—are well documented across countless studies, some of which are referenced here in this book. What you will find in the following pages is meant for informational purposes only and should not be considered gospel. We recommend that you always consult your doctor before embarking on any plan to lose weight to ensure it's best for you.

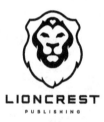

LIONCREST
PUBLISHING

CONTENTS

PART III
HERE'S WHAT WORKS

INTRODUCTION

I could have died. That fact was made clear by the serious faces around me and the urgent efforts to get me into the operating room, *STAT!*

But I wasn't thinking about dying.

Maybe if I had thought about the seriousness of my condition, I would have been scared. Maybe, as I lay strapped on the gurney watching the ceiling tiles speed past, I would have been sad, fearful of never seeing my family again. But there was no room for fear. I was too angry.

I wasn't supposed to be there. I was supposed to be heading out to have lunch with a friend before playing a few games on the tennis court later that afternoon. I was supposed to be standing upright and feeling great, joking with my own patients as I helped them improve their health. Instead, an anesthetist was prepping to knock me out for heart surgery. How was that possible? I'd done everything I was supposed to do to prevent something like this!

Sure, I'd gained a little weight after college. And yes, while I focused on my career, building my practice, the extra pounds continued to plague me. But I was someone who'd been practicing what he preached for years. I took care of myself the way I encouraged my patients to take care of themselves by eating right and exercising. So it just didn't make sense to me when, at the age of forty-nine, I landed in the OR still twenty-five pounds overweight. Granted, my triglycerides were high. But six out of my seven siblings could say the same thing. Clearly, there was a genetic tendency at play here —yet none of *them* had a heart attack at such a young age. Only I did. Me. Why? How?

When I found out my triglycerides were high back in the late 1980s, I did what was recommended and changed my diet. I became a vegetarian. But wouldn't you know it? My triglycerides raised even higher! That wasn't what I expected at all. Even worse, the new diet did nothing to help me lose weight. And that's when my adventures with dieting began.

I tried everything. Usually, I'd lose around six pounds at the get-go, but the second I veered off the plan for a minor infringement—say one slice of pizza as a celebratory meal—I'd put those pounds back on overnight. Now *that* certainly didn't make sense to me. I mean, never had I eaten a piece of pizza that weighed six pounds! How was that kind of weight gain even possible?

I tried fasting, sometimes for as long as five days. And every January, I would do a twenty-one-day cleanse that would take off a little more than my regular six pounds, but by March—when I'd return to a clean and healthy diet of recommended calories—I'd be right back to where I was on New Year's Eve.

On top of all the dieting, I exercised—a lot! I was, and still am, very active. As I do now, I rode my bike, played tennis, golfed, and participated in many other activities on a regular basis. Again, I was doing everything right. So why didn't I lose any weight? Why didn't my triglycerides go down? Why, instead of lobbing a ball over the net with my backhand, was I on an operating table? What was wrong with my body?

WHY IS IT SO HARD TO LOSE WEIGHT?

If you're reading this, you've probably asked similar questions about your body. Why can't I lose weight? Why is this so hard? And, whether it's just a few pounds or a hundred to shed, Dan and I would place money on you having tried at least one diet to lose it. We'll go a step further and bet that whatever you tried didn't work. If our guesses are correct, don't think it's because we can read minds or anything. We just happen to know the statistics.

In a survey that spanned three years, the CDC discovered that almost half of the American adult population had tried to lose weight within the twelve months prior to responding to the survey,[1] and most of them did it through dieting. Unfortunately, though, studies from UCLA[2] and others have repeatedly demonstrated that *up to two-thirds of the people who do manage to lose weight on their diets wind up gaining it back* (as well as some extra pounds, because who doesn't like a bonus?).

Before you think those statistics make losing weight sound hopeless, read on!

We're here to tell you it *is* possible to lose weight. It doesn't matter how long you've been struggling with it, how much you have to lose, or why you need to lose it. We *know* you can lose it because we've helped many people from all walks of life do just that.

We've helped women whose children are in their teens finally lose that last fifteen pounds of pregnancy weight. We've helped athletes, both male and female, lose the extra layer of fat they thought was impossible to shed. We've helped mature adults lose the excess pounds that they'd slowly put on through the years despite trying a multitude of diet plans. And we've helped young adults who are tired of struggling to be OK with their weight as they focus on building successful careers achieve a body that is healthy and slim. Some of our clients only wanted to lose ten pounds, but we've had a few who successfully lost a hundred pounds.

What makes us so sure about our plan, though, is how personal it is to us. Not only has it worked for me, but our plan has also helped our family members and loved ones finally achieve and maintain a healthy weight.

Even better: just about everyone is happy. No one is hungry. And possibly more important, no one is terrified of donuts after they lose the weight.

We've been so successful because we understand that losing weight is more than just counting calories and fitness training. It's about discovering what *your* unique body needs and then custom tailoring the right approach for you to get those needs met.

SO WHAT DOES IT TAKE TO LOSE WEIGHT?

Despite being so angry, I can't say how much I appreciate the good doctors who took care of me in the operating room that day. Apparently, I had a 90 percent blockage in my heart that required two stents. Oh, and my triglycerides were at 1,100. For perspective, healthy levels are 150 or below. So you could say I was a super-achiever cardiac patient that day—not everyone manages to reach such high numbers. However, I was more than a little demoralized by the situation. I couldn't even face my friends and family in the waiting room who were there to support me. I felt like I'd failed them—and me.

However, the timing of my heart attack couldn't have been more appropriate. Would you believe the day I was discharged was on New Year's Eve? That's right, it was the time of year when we prepare for fresh starts and are eager to make good on resolutions to improve our lives. When we are supposed to be excited and hopeful. I wanted to tap into that excitement and energy because, as my wife and I exited those hospital doors, it was obvious to me I needed to make some improvements. But where was I to start? And what would I do? It seemed as if I had already tried everything I could think of to lose weight and get control of my body chemistry. Yet look where it got me!

I wasn't ready to go back to treating my patients yet, so I took a month off from work and went to Florida with the intention of recuperating and wrapping my head around just what, exactly, had happened to me. I became a vegan and started running. Within nine months, I ran my first marathon. But guess what? If I lost any weight at all, it was negligible. And my triglycerides? They weren't overachieving quite so much, but they were still not in a great place.

Three years later, I was still a vegan . . . and still overweight. So, when my wife and I bumped into an old colleague of mine who told me about his new method of weight loss, something that I'd never heard of, I was intrigued. While his plan seemed a bit far-fetched in that it required using technology to measure things like micronutrients, I liked the science behind it. So I gave it a shot, thinking what did I have to lose?

Apparently, I had twenty-five pounds to lose! Which I did in twenty days while cutting my triglyceride levels in half.

Six months later, the weight remained off and my triglycerides were within normal ranges. Eleven years later, I've maintained a healthy range with my blood chemistry *and* I'm still at a good weight, despite treating myself to some good pizza, celebratory or not.

I have since worked with Dan to overhaul and perfect that original plan to make it the most comprehensive and user-friendly approach to weight loss we could create. Now, it is the protocol we use at our *re:vitalize weight loss* clinics and with our remote clients. It is also what you'll learn about in this book—and what we believe will help get you started on your own weight loss journey, where you will learn to fear no food.

In Part 1, we talk about the various factors at play that make it not only easy to gain weight but almost impossible *not* to. We begin in Chapter 1 by discussing how stress and hormonal imbalances are at the root of weight issues for many people. Unfortunately, unless those folks address the physiological impact of stress or rebalance their hormones, they may never find a way to lose weight. What is fortunate, though, is that there are plans that can help them do just that. It's a matter of figuring out what *your* particular body needs, then applying a nutritional strategy to fulfil those needs.

With what seems like an unending list of diets anyone can try, you would think it would be easy to find the right one for you. However, as Chapter 2 discusses, not all diets are created equally. And while there will always be a few people who can and do succeed on each one of them, most people will not. Even worse—for many, the rebound effect will add on more pounds! So instead of giving you a diet, we're going to talk about what a good nutritional plan should look like and how to fit it into your life.

The thing is, changing your diet often requires a massive overhaul in your behavior and thoughts. And, as with any other strong habit, adopting a new lifestyle around food is daunting and downright hard, particularly at first. Knowing that might make it difficult to even find the courage to start. And then, when you finally do get going, there's always the potential to hit a snag that tempts you to give up before you lose the amount you wanted to.

So, to help you overcome those fears and the temptation to quit, Part 2 begins with a little motivation to keep up the efforts. In Chapter 3, we talk about how losing weight can have a positive impact on just about every area of your life. By losing excess weight and maintaining a healthy one, you'll feel a boost in your mood and energy that creates a positive carry-over effect throughout your life. I can't tell you how many patients have told us that one of the best parts about losing weight is that, because they were happier and more uplifting to be around, their relationships with their loved ones improved. Not only that, but their love lives improved. Overall, losing weight increased their quality of life.

If you need more help in the motivation area, and many of us do, Chapter 4 discusses how positive psychology can go a long way toward helping you stay on your nutritional plan. You'll discover a few proven tactics around the way you talk to and about yourself makes it easier to find success with your weight loss goals.

And, if you're struggling with a medical condition on top of your weight problem, you may find Chapter 5 inspiring. Many primary care doctors and other medical specialists refer patients to us, and many of those patients are delighted to discover they can stop taking medications for type 2 diabetes, hypertension, cholesterol, heart-burn, thyroid issues, and other diseases simply because they were able to lose weight. And for those who have to remain on medica-tion, most find great improvements in their levels of inflammation and energy.

Part 3 is where you'll finally learn the methods and strategies behind our weight loss program. In Chapter 6, we provide some tools for you to implement at any time to get started on your weight loss journey. Then in Chapter 7, you'll learn about the micronutrients in your foods and how, by ensuring you get adequate amounts of them, you can stave off cravings. Here we'll also provide you with some tricks of the trade that will help you make better choices to support your slim-down.

In Chapter 8, we talk about how high-tech instruments can identify your particular bio-chemical needs to really home in on the right whole foods and nutrients for your unique body. And Chapter 9 reminds you that there is no need to go it alone. It's important to have an accountability buddy or coach helping you every step of the way as you put a plan into action. Just as Pavarotti, the famous opera singer, continued to have a voice coach his entire life, you will find that keeping a support structure for your weight loss is an invaluable lifelong tool.

Understanding
Body Composition Analysis

In each chapter, we'll tell you a little bit about some of our patients, which includes their body composition analysis (BCA) numbers. At re:vitalize, we consider the BCA one of our most important insights because it provides an in-depth, real-time assessment of your current health status and your progress. Through Resonant Frequency Technology, we get biometric data that enables us to create the perfect program for each of our patients to lose weight. We measure:

- Body Mass Index (BMI): a standard height-to-weight ratio that is often used to determine health risks related to obesity (but as you'll discover later, this statistic isn't one we put too much faith in).

- Body Fat Percentage: just what it sounds like: it's the proportion of your body that consists of fat.

- Body Fat Mass: the actual weight of the fat on your body.

- Metabolic Age: the number we get after comparing all the body composition facts together. The lower your age, the faster your metabolism.

- Visceral Fat Rating: this is the amount of fat that is in the internal abdominal cavity and surrounding organs. The more fat you have surrounding your vital organs, the higher your chances of having heart disease, high blood pressure, type 2 diabetes, and other diseases.

- Basal Metabolic Rate: this tells us about how many calories your body uses to maintain normal functioning while resting.

- Body Water Percentage: gives us an idea of how much water is in your cells, which is an indicator of true hydration.

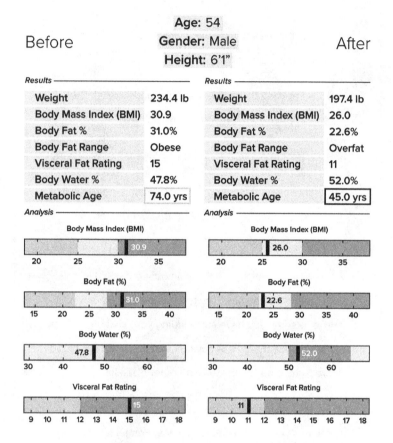

Age: 54
Gender: Male
Height: 6'1"

Before

Results ————————————————

Weight	234.4 lb
Body Mass Index (BMI)	30.9
Body Fat %	31.0%
Body Fat Range	Obese
Visceral Fat Rating	15
Body Water %	47.8%
Metabolic Age	74.0 yrs

Analysis ————————————————

After

Results ————————————————

Weight	197.4 lb
Body Mass Index (BMI)	26.0
Body Fat %	22.6%
Body Fat Range	Overfat
Visceral Fat Rating	11
Body Water %	52.0%
Metabolic Age	45.0 yrs

Analysis ————————————————

Chapter 10 will end the book by providing you with a few recipes for healthy eating that many of our clients have found useful and delicious on their own weight loss journey. Along the way, we hope you enjoy our Doc and Dan Do's—quick tips and tricks Dan and I use on a regular basis that help us maintain the weight we are at.

WHY DO WE BELIEVE IN THIS PROGRAM?

This program works. It's that simple. My own success with it inspired me to open a clinic to help others reach their weight loss goals. Although I had a thriving wellness practice already, I knew I wanted to expand my services to include this program. And I knew I wanted Dan to be my partner.

Not only is Dan my son-in-law, but he has the heart and insight needed to build a caring and professional business team. While Dan himself never really suffered from a weight problem, many people in his family did. He grew up watching them deal with the day-to-day frustration of being overweight. And he saw first-hand the negative impact being heavy has on a person's quality of life.

Dan also has a diverse abundance of life experiences. Shortly after college, he played rugby in Scotland. At the ready to stay in peak condition during that time, he became a supplement and exercise guinea pig, in a constant attempt to maintain and improve his health. When he returned to the States, Dan and my daughter, Danae, went to the Dominican Republic to serve with a non-profit doing education and economic development work. They lived there for five years in a mountainous agricultural area where fresh fruits and vegetables grew in abundance. Dan couldn't help but notice how the people he served there, although monetarily poor, were in pretty good shape thanks to the wealth of fresh produce around them. They ate a healthy, plant-based diet and had a very active lifestyle.

Having always been passionate about fitness, health, and nutrition, when he returned to the States, Dan went on to receive two board certifications in holistic nutrition. Like me, he had a tendency to look beyond the status quo weight loss and health and was greatly interested in discovering new science-based approaches. However, Dan was a bit skeptical of the program at first. But after he watched his mother drop thirty pounds and reduce her metabolic age to the mid-thirties (when she was fifty-five), he became a believer. And when he realized she was keeping the weight off, and how happy that made her, he just knew he had to be part of such a positive and powerful practice.

BUT ENOUGH ABOUT US

This book is about and for you. It's about what *you* need to know to get a handle on *your* weight.

We can't say it will all be easy. Particularly at the beginning, our plan can be a little tough. But once you make it through to the other side, once you attain the weight you want, you will not ever fear food again.

We know life is about more than just being thin. We all celebrate good times, special events, and family traditions around piles of food, which is often fat- and sugar-laden. What good is being skinny if you have to ban yourself from partaking in those good times ever again?

While no one will be able to eat chocolate cake for breakfast, lunch, and dinner every day for the rest of their life, everyone should be able to eat a normal amount food they love without worrying about gaining everything back. That's not just our philosophy—it's what we teach *and* practice. Once you heal your metabolism and learn what foods work best for your body, you'll be able to eat what you want without gaining weight. And should you ever gain a few extra pounds—say, overindulging on an extended holiday vacation—you'll have the tools you need to lose it again.

If you're ready to hear more about our method of weight loss, turn the page and start learning how you, too, can fear no food by finding the right dieting method for you.

PART I

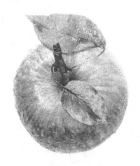

LET'S GET READY

CHAPTER 1

WHAT'S GOING ON WITH MY BODY?

"Ever since (fill in the blank), I can't lose weight!"

Whether it's *had a baby, changed careers, hit forty, had back surgery,* or something else, we can't tell you how many of our clients begin a sentence with those words during their first consultation with us. They say it with justifiable frustration and anger, and sometimes even with sadness. Because the truth is sometimes things happen in our lives that sort of flip a switch in our bodies and make it difficult for us to lose weight.

Sometimes the switch happens quickly—like after a car accident or sudden loss of a job—and we immediately start gaining noticeable amounts of weight. But other times, the switch happens over time, and we don't notice exactly when it began, until we reflect back on our lives and realize, *Oh yeah, you know what? The weight gain started after we had the last baby.*

Gaining slowly over time is how one of our clients experienced his weight troubles. The crazy thing is his switch happened to be exercise.

Brian knew something was wrong with his body. For years he'd been training hard for triathlon competitions where he did very well. In fact, he had reached a level of fame in that community because he frequently put up "Personal Best" records at international championships. A Personal Best record is when you prove you are faster, stronger, and an overall better athlete then you were at any prior event. He became well known for being fit, fast, and strong, and had a large number of people following him on social media. Up until a few years ago, he looked fit, fast, and strong, too. But then his body started to change. He felt it and noticed it—and unfortunately, the folks on social media made comments about how they noticed it, too.

Even worse, he felt terrible. He'd spent years pushing through being tired, and now he was completely exhausted. His body just couldn't train any more—the energy wasn't there, and it was taking him much longer to recover after a competition. When he thought about it, he realized he was spending more time in pain than out of it. He wasn't sleeping well. And, perhaps what made the least sense to him, he was gaining fat.

No matter what he did, he gained weight.

Cut calories? Regardless of what kind of limits he put on himself, the weight continued to creep upward. So he tried the opposite: he added more calories, thinking perhaps his metabolism had slowed down from cutting too many out. Nope. He still gained weight.

Work out harder? More? Was that even possible? No matter what he did, this former picture of health and fitness continued to get heavier and lose energy.

By the time the COVID pandemic forced many communities into lockdown, Brian had hit the proverbial wall. He was so tired and out of shape he felt a secret sense of relief that he had to stay indoors and out of the gym. Now he had a "legitimate" excuse to take time off from training. Maybe his social media followers wouldn't think it so shocking that he was packing on weight. Even better, maybe he could figure out what was going on with his body.

Dan was able to sum up Brian's problem within minutes: this world-class athlete's biochemistry was completely out of whack due to the physical and mental stress he was enduring. *Out of whack* isn't exactly a medical term, but we don't think there is a better way to describe what was going on in Brian's body. It's a phenomenon we see with many of our clients, and not all of them are athletes but from all walks of life.

Client Body Composition Biodata: Before and After Results

Brian	27 yo | 5' 7" | Male		
	Before	**After**	**Difference**
Weight	181.4	155.2	-26.2
BMI Change/Improvement			-4.1
Body Fat % Lost			-10.7%
Visceral Fat Rating Improvement			-5.1
Cellular Hydration Improvement[1]			+6%
Metabolic Improvement[2]			-34 yrs

[1] Change in body water %
[2] As measured by metabolic age reversal/improvement

For many people, the reason they cannot lose weight no matter how hard they try is that their body is out of balance (whack), usually due to stress. Stress really does a number on our hormones, which subsequently does a number on our metabolism, which increases the numbers on the scale.

HOW DOES
STRESS IMPACT WEIGHT?

To understand how and why stress makes us gain weight, we need to look at how certain hormones work in your body. I promise not to make this book too heavy with medical jargon and the science behind your body chemistry. I know you came here for help losing weight, not for a biochemistry lesson. But I do think it's important that you understand some fundamentals so that you'll understand why Dan and I believe in, and find success in, our approach to weight loss.

There are several hormones that impact your weight, but the three that we think are the most important are leptin, ghrelin, and cortisol.

Leptin and Ghrelin, Your Drive-in and Diner Hormones

Our fat cells aren't exactly lazy. Among other things, they work hard to produce leptin, which is kind of interesting when you realize that the job of leptin is to prevent you from accumulating too much fat. It does that by signaling that full feeling you get from a meal. You start eating, your body checks in with your fat levels that say, "We need *this much* energy," and when you hit that point in your food, leptin comes in and hangs the "closed for lunch" sign on the stomach (unless, of course, it's dinner or breakfast . . . it has several signs).

Working in the opposite direction, ghrelin is a hormone your stomach produces that tells you it's time to find an open diner. Ghrelin makes us feel hungry or like we want to eat. After experiencing a stressor, our stomach sends out the ghrelin alert to make you want to eat. Why? As you'll soon see in the discussion on the liver, when you are stressed, your body primes itself to use a lot of energy. After a stressor, your stomach thinks you need to replenish your fuel levels.

Often ghrelin is what's behind stress eating. Ever wonder why you don't crave celery when you're stressed? It's crunchy and you can make it salty, so why not that over potato chips? That's because ghrelin knows the best and quickest way to give you fuel is through fast-acting carbohydrates like sugar, flour, white rice, and starchy vegetables. But it also knows that the fast-acting part will be used up and something needs to follow it—what better chaser than fatty foods?

So leptin says, "No more food," while ghrelin says, "More, please." When life happens and stress piles up, those hormones go out of balance. Ghrelin puts your refrigerator on speed-dial, and leptin does its best to keep up.[3] After leptin is over-ridden for a period of time, your body can begin to think it's not a hormone you need to pay attention to, and you develop something called leptin resistance— you no longer receive those signals saying you've had enough.[4] So you eat and eat some more, never feeling satisfied.

The thing is, leptin resistance has another cause, the third hormone we need to talk about: cortisol. And that requires a discussion about our livers.

Liver: Your Emotional Baggage Check-in Point

Your liver is a pretty amazing organ. It helps fight bacteria and viruses that can make you sick. It makes the majority of the stuff that's necessary for your blood to clot. It produces bile that is needed to digest your food. And—perhaps one of the most important things your liver does—it removes toxins you may have ingested along with whatever you happened to eat or drink.

Similarly, when you breathe in pollution or absorb chemicals through your skin, your bloodstream will take those toxins to your liver to get rid of them. Most of the time your liver does a pretty good job of handling all of those responsibilities very well. However, when you experience stress, most of that stuff comes to a screeching halt.

It's not that your liver quits working when you're under stress. It just changes focus. When you experience fear, worry, or other negative emotions that are indicators of stress, your liver teams up with your adrenal glands—two little glands that sit atop each of your kidneys —to create part of your fight, flight, or freeze response. You may have heard of that before: it's what happens inside your body when you experience something that causes fear or stress.

In short, the flight part of that stress response is when your body kicks everything into gear to help you escape a stressor. The liver starts producing glucose (sugar) and fats (in the form of cholesterol) to provide the fuel you need to run far and long. The adrenals, meanwhile, produce cortisol, which shuts down bodily functions that it deems are not needed during an emergency (like digestion). At the same time, cortisol amps up your energy levels by assisting that sugar to get into your bloodstream (among other processes we don't need to go into now).

The fight, flight, or freeze response is the perfect thing to help you escape from wild tigers or bears. In fact, that's why it's there—to give you the energy to escape. But your body cannot tell the difference between a typical bad day and a wild tiger chasing after you.

When you are running late for work because your child has a fever and you need to make alternate day-care arrangements, you're worrying about your kid and being late for work, but your body is fueling you to escape a grizzly bear. Then, after you drop your child off at the sitter and get stuck in a traffic jam, you're stewing about and fretting about the inconvenience, but your body is giving you more fuel. And you can probably guess what happens when you get to work and your boss harangues you for being late and you have to deal with the myriad "emergencies" there, whether it's a jammed printer or a client firing you.

Unfortunately, things don't usually end there, do they? After work, there's more traffic before you get home to realize, yet again, you can't help your oldest one with his math homework because who understands that stuff anymore? The evening news upsets you, which you try to hide as you call your mom to see how her physical therapy is going. Next thing you know, you need to sit down to sort the mail and pay some bills—but ugh! The cat just threw up again! Does he intentionally aim for the carpet?

Your body simply can't tell those tense moments of "the daily grind" from a grizzly bear ripping open your back door to find your secret stash of Reese's Cups. So it keeps pumping out the energy to help you deal with a life-endangering threat . . . all day, every day. And our bodies were never meant to be in a constant state of stress.

We are designed to experience stress momentarily, then use up all that excess energy (sugar and cholesterol) to escape whatever is scaring us. Think about it—when you're being chased by a wild animal, you need that fuel to run. So what happens when you're under chronic stress and never get to run to the safety of the cave? Instead of burning off that sugar and cholesterol, you wind up with an excess of it that gets stored as fat somewhere in your body. And the belly, hips, and thighs are easy storage places.

But that's only part one. Remember, your liver cannot multitask when it's stressed. So its entire toxin-cleaning factory shuts down in order to deal with your stressors. And it does so at the same time that cortisol shuts down your digestive system (or at least slows it, because the last thing you need to do when you're running away from a grizzly bear is to make a pit stop).

The consequences here are twofold: one, when you don't properly digest your food, it ferments in your stomach and you don't get the nutrients you need from it. That drains you and can cause malnourishment, fuzzy thinking, and feelings of weakness. Second, you now have toxins in your body that your liver can't handle, and they need to be put somewhere. The good news is your blood stream knows exactly where to look: those handy storage places called fat cells. The more toxins in need of disposing, the more fat is made on your body. This fat is stuff your body is resistant to releasing because it doesn't want those toxins just floating around where they can potentially do damage, so it is not easily burned off.

Now Brian's situation probably makes more sense. His body started putting on fat thanks to the constant stress of exercise and training. Most likely, his stewing over and worrying about his social media image compounded the physical stress.

This may even make sense of the spare tire around our middle many of us find in middle age: all those years of working up the corporate ladder eventually take their toll. And do I even need to discuss parenting stress? Do any of us think we'll survive teaching our teenagers to drive? Then when we do, do we ever stop worrying about them out there on the road? No wonder they give us both white hair *and* a muffin top!

But so far, I've only talked about chronic stress. Acute stress can be just as bad for us, mostly because we don't let them go. A minor car accident where we walk away unharmed only lasts a few seconds, but we often revisit the fear as we tell everyone we know about it or reflect back on it as we drive past that spot again and again.

Being on the receiving end of a nasty comment from a grocery store clerk that makes us feel victimized somehow. It becomes something we hold onto when we vent to our partners and complain about it on Facebook, where your friends chime in and confirm you were being verbally attacked, and it never dies. Unless we can learn to let such instances roll off of us like water off a duck's back—becoming something we shake off and forget about or something we process by going for a good run—they will often wind up manifesting as excess weight.

OUR TOXIC LIVES

Even if you do go for a run, though, the weight may not come off if your stress is chronic. Remember, your liver isn't detoxing if it's dealing with stressors. So all those toxins that you've been exposed to, that your blood has stored in your fat, are still there waiting until your liver is ready to deal with them. And your body will resist releasing that fat because it doesn't want those toxins floating around in it. That's right: you can perfect the duck-shaking-water-off attitude, chill out, and relax for the rest of your life, but you won't lose excess weight until you get those toxins out of your body!

You may be wondering how your food could have toxins. We live in a first-world country and buy food in the grocery store! How can it be toxic?

Doc and Dan Do: buy organic whenever possible. Sure, it may be more expensive, but when you think about your long-term health, you'll see it's worth it!

By toxins, I'm referring to the pesticides, herbicides, and fungicides that are sprayed onto the fruits and vegetables we eat. Yes, they are deemed "safe" by regulatory agencies, but that safety rating is often found to be debatable by many in the natural health communities. Besides, regardless of whether they are safe for us, our bodies don't recognize them as nourishing foods; therefore, they don't believe they are safe, which is why our liver says they must go. But toxins from foods aren't all your liver needs to manage.

Look up the ingredients in your personal care items in the Skin Deep database the Environmental Working Group[5] has put together; you may be shocked and dismayed by the potential damage they can be doing to your body. Just look at what a few of the ingredients in this shampoo have the potential to do (I won't reveal the name of it, but it is a very popular shampoo sold across the country):

- Coal tar: a known human carcinogen(!) and respiratory tract toxicant; this ingredient is classified as being a "high human healthy priority" and is *expected* to be harmful![6]

- Propylparaben: this is an endocrine disruptor (something that messes with our hormones), particularly with male sex hormones, and is a cause of allergies and dermatitis.[7]

- Fragrance: this is probably one of the most common ingredients not just in shampoos but in many personal care products like lotions, makeup, and body washes. Unfortunately, many chemicals fall under this category, and they can cause contact dermatitis or worsen asthma.[8]

I could go on and on about the dangers in the products we use on our bodies, then launch into a discussion about all the cleaning chemicals we use in our homes and the outdoor environmental pollution surrounding us. But that would mean writing another book, and you're only here to learn about losing weight.

The key takeaway here is to realize that everything we are exposed to can and does absorb into our skin and get breathed into our lungs. Our livers have a tough job to clean it all out. And as you now know, if we're stressed so much that our hormones are working to make energy (fat), our liver just can't get rid of it all. The only answer is to store it in the fat.

Actually, that's not the *only* answer. You can also detox, which is a primary concern for us in our nutritional strategy for weight loss.

DETOX—IT'S NOT JUST FOR ROCK STARS ANYMORE

Our program stresses clean vegetables and fruits, which means organic produce. The proteins you eat also need to be clean. That translates to free-range, organic poultry; grass-fed (or grass finished) beef and bison; and wild-caught fish. At the beginning of our plan, we put an emphasis on eating only a minimum of fat so that your body is forced to burn the fat it's been storing on you for fuel. But you need to do that safely, with appropriate minerals and vitamins to support that burn and help get the toxins out of you.

The specific minerals and vitamins you take will vary depending on your unique biological markers (as we'll discuss in Chapter 8). However, there are plenty of things you can do to help your body naturally detox:

- Chill. Do what you can to relax and decompress from stress. At the very minimum, take time at the end of each day to reflect on your life and spend a few minutes in gratitude, as described in the free resources at http://www.fearno foodbook.com/. If your stress is intense, get help. Whether it's learning meditation or yoga, joining a support group, speaking with clergy, or seeing a therapist, it's important you get help dealing with whatever it is life is throwing at you. We all heal and recuperate better when we have a support structure in place.

- Stay hydrated! Having enough water in your body will help flush out toxins.

- Get some sleep. Did you know when you sleep, a mechanism in your brain makes your brain cells shrink so it can flush toxins out? Sleep is one of the easiest ways to detox![9]

- Eat clean! Abstain from sugar, refined carbohydrates, alcohol, and all forms of junk food. Whatever junk you put in your body will only clog it up and work against your natural ability to detox.

- Go green! We encourage people to eat a pound of vegetables every day. And the best ones to help with detoxification are asparagus, broccoli, kale, artichokes, spinach, and collard greens. These green vegetables are packed with nutrients that your body uses to bind toxins and make them water soluble so you can eliminate them.

- Indulge in avocados. Not only do these wonders have healthy fats in them (and taste great grilled), but they are also loaded with antioxidants that help your body detox.

- Get regular with fiber from beets. The betaine in these red roots also aids the liver's detox processes, and their fiber is in the form of pectin, which helps clear the toxins out of your body.

You see? Detox doesn't have to involve starving yourself as you live on lemon juice and cayenne pepper or doing something else equally intense. It's really a matter of incorporating some strategies that we should all be doing anyway if we want to be healthy in general. Yes, there are particular supplements that can also help your body's detox pathways work even better, but that is something you could discuss during a consultation with one of our nutritionists or weight loss coaches. Most of us can get great detox benefits from incorporating the above ideas into our lives.

Now that you know *why* it's so hard to lose weight, it's time to choose a particular strategy to do so. But with so many diet plans, meal plans, nutritional plans, and wellness plans, how do you pick? Well, Dan and I have a few ideas about that, and it's what we'll talk about next.

CHAPTER 2

ALL DIETS WORK— FOR THE RIGHT PERSON

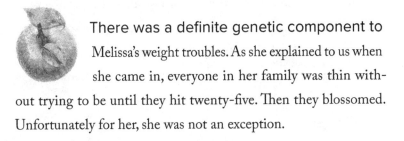

There was a definite genetic component to Melissa's weight troubles. As she explained to us when she came in, everyone in her family was thin without trying to be until they hit twenty-five. Then they blossomed. Unfortunately for her, she was not an exception.

Melissa didn't have a care about her weight for a long while. Up through her early twenties, she ate whatever she wanted, whenever she wanted, and as much of it as she wanted, yet still remained slim and strong. But when she came into our office at the age of thirty-three, she was at a weight that depressed her. In her wedding photos, she sees the body she had when she was thirty pounds lighter, and it makes her sad and frustrated. She wasn't even trying to be thin back then!

Granted, she now has a sedentary job sitting at a desk for eight hours every day, but she did walk the parking lot for an hour at lunch every day and ran several times a week because she was training for a 5K event. When asked about her diet, she explained that she primarily ate a little fish and a bunch of rabbit food: salads and veggies. She did add some egg and avocado to her salads and some light vinaigrette, but not enough to maintain the weight she was at.

It was clear to Dan when he spoke to her that Melissa needed to reboot her metabolism. After doing a body composition analysis of her with the technology in our *re:vitalize weight loss* office, we discovered her metabolism was that of a woman a couple of *decades* older than she was! That meant her internal furnace wasn't burning fuel the way it should for a thirty-three-year-old woman. Her body was taking in the calories but not properly burning them.

The next question was why?

For Melissa, a full bioscan (which we'll explain in Chapter 8) revealed she had some nutritional imbalances. Various levels of vitamins, minerals, and micronutrients were off in her body. Part of that may have been a genetic tendency, but the other part goes back to various stressors in her life. Remember, stress slows down your digestion so you are not able to get all the nutrients you need, and if you're eating a diet as most Americans do that is high in refined carbohydrates and low in fruits and vegetables, you're barely getting those nutrients to begin with.

Client Body Composition Biodata: Before and After Results

Melissa	33 yo	5' 4"	Female			
	Before	After	Difference
Weight	190.2	174	-16.2
BMI Change/Improvement			-2.7
Visceral Fat Rating Improvement			-1.3
Cellular Hydration Improvement[1]			+1.3%
Metabolic Improvement[2]			-32 yrs

[1] Change in body water %
[2] As measured by metabolic age reversal/improvement

That last part wasn't Melissa's current problem, but after digging in a little more in her history, she admitted she ate like a typical teenager and young adult "back in the day," when vegetables were not her top choice.

The good news for Melissa—and everybody—is that her biological age could be reset. It was a matter of ensuring adequate hydration and feeding her the right supplements to get her nutrient levels in balance again.

We put Melissa on our nutritional plan and suggested specific supplements, and she dropped those extra thirty pounds. But that's not all. Because we reset her metabolic age, she discovered she can (and does) eat whatever she wants yet again because she now has the metabolism of her youth to burn it all off.

YOU'RE UNIQUE, JUST LIKE ME!

Age is just one factor that influences your metabolism. Other factors include activity levels, habitual food choices, medical conditions, and body size. Let's take a quick peek at some real-life scenarios we've successfully worked with that truly depict how different we are:

- Client One is a former NBA star who played on the court with the likes of Michael Jordan and Charles Barkley. He's six feet, seven inches tall and still pretty active in his pastimes. But he's not as active as he was when he was young, and he still has the appetite of his youth. He's on TV and radio each week, so he feels some pressure to maintain his physique. The last thing he wants is some fan of his former rival to poke fun at his weight on Twitter!

- Client Two, meanwhile, could be considered Client One's opposite. She's five feet, two inches tall, menopausal, and has a fairly sedentary lifestyle aside from walking three or four days a week. She's been on a variety of diet plans, saying she's "done everything under the sun" from bars and shakes to diet pills and human chorionic gonadotropin (HCG) shots. She also tried Jenny Craig and Weight Watchers, all to no avail. Sure, she'd lose a few pounds with each plan at the beginning, but she quickly puts it back on without even trying.

- Client Three is a middle-aged executive male. He's six feet tall, solidly built, and relatively active. He hikes and lifts weights a few days a week and sees a personal trainer on the days in between. At one point, he had to have knee surgery, and ever since, he's had trouble maintaining his weight.

- Client Four is a high school girl on summer vacation. She's five feet, six inches tall and plays four hours of tennis at camp every day. She has a robust social life, which means she eats out with her friends *a lot* and, despite all the tennis, it's showing.

Just a quick glance at those profiles will tell you they are all in different phases of their lives. Their motivations to lose weight are different. They all have different backgrounds and energy usage patterns, and most likely, they all have had different stressors in their lives. On top of that, our metabolism naturally changes as we age, and no two people experience the identical rate of change.

Taking in all of those differences, which diet plan do you think they should choose?

EENIE, MEENIE, MINEY, MO!

With so many diet plans out there, sometimes it seems as if all you need to do is just pick one at random. After all, most of them have science and statistics to back up their claims, and all have plenty of anecdotal evidence. If you didn't know better, it might be tempting to pick one via *eenie, meenie, miney, mo!*

But if it were that simple, you wouldn't be reading this book, right? And now that you know stress and hormones are such big influencers on your weight, as well as your toxic load, you probably realize losing weight is much more complex than a matter of calories-in-calories-out.

> *"We should be personalizing diets and not just trying to squeeze everyone into the same shoe size."*
>
> **TIM SPECTER**, epidemiologist and professor at King's College in London

Before we go further, I thought it would be helpful to look at a few of the most common approaches to dieting out there today. These are the ones we hear about most from our clients who have tried them. I think when you look at their pros and cons, you'll realize that none of them will work for everyone. If you're not interested in all the detailed pros and cons of the various approaches outlined here (or have already tried your hand at many and don't want to relive them) feel free to skip ahead to learn the six questions everyone should ask before starting any weight loss program.

Bars, Shakes, and Prepackaged Foods

These types of plans provide the food required in prepackaged meals, bars, and shakes. In that sense, they make it easy to eat the limited number of calories they prescribe.

Pros

- They usually provide wonderful online or in-person support to help you figure out your target weight and to keep you motivated. We believe that personal touch from someone who understands what you're going through and has the know-how to support you is integral for any life change—diet or otherwise.

- Their plans are easy to follow, in part because they provide the food. And when they don't provide the food, they do have simple recipes, food tips, and exercise guides.

- The number of calories is already counted for you, so there is no need for guesswork.

Cons

- Many of the meals contain (what we consider) questionable ingredients that are highly processed and sometimes artificial. We believe foods like this are "too far out of the kitchen," meaning we don't consider them "real" foods that provide the nutrition your body craves.

- There is a lack of vegetables and fruit.

- Many of the shakes contain quite a bit of sugar.

- The meals are light on fiber as well as calories. In fact, many are so light on calories that some of the items labeled as snacks and desserts have the same calorie count as those labeled as meals.

Keto

"Keto" is short for ketogenic. It's a low-carbohydrate, moderate-protein, and high-fat diet that intentionally puts your body in a state of ketosis in order to burn fat.

See, your body converts everything you eat into glucose (sugar) to burn as fuel. When you feed it refined carbohydrates, no converting is necessary. It just uses that energy if it needs it, and then it stores what it doesn't need as fat. If you do not eat enough carbohydrates to satisfy your need for fuel, your body must then burn off the fat you have in reserves. So it converts that fat into glucose, and when it does that, ketones are produced as a by-product, which also supply energy. You achieve ketosis when your body uses the ketones for fuel.

Pros

- Weight loss is the biggest pro. Not only does it come from ketosis, but also from reducing calorie intake by eliminating food groups.

- People feel less hungry because fatty foods take a longer time to break down in the body.

- No more low-fat! Many people love the keto diet because they get to eat all the high-fat foods they enjoy with little restrictions—red meat, fatty fish, nuts, cheese, butter, and even bacon—all while losing weight.

Cons

- It's difficult to sustain. Because of the stringent food restrictions, many find the keto diet hard to stick to.

- Nutrient deficiency from the restricted list of acceptable foods means you don't receive the nutrients—vitamins, minerals, and fibers—that you get from fresh fruits, legumes, vegetables, and whole grains. Due to these deficiencies, people report feeling foggy and tired.

- Food obsession can result from the need to monitor your intake so closely, which can lead to psychological distress such as shame and binge eating. The restrictions on types of food allowed compounds the obsession and can encourage bingeing, which often leads to guilt, which then leads back to restriction in a continuous cycle.

- The high-fat nature of the diet includes a number of bad or unhealthy fats, which could have a negative impact on heart health, as explained in this video: https://tinyurl.com/StopDoingKeto.

- Finding ongoing true support can be hard. Sure, there are numerous Facebook groups with gurus leading them, but are they qualified to answer all your questions and provide the motivation to stay on course? Possibly, but possibly not.

Vegan Diet

A vegan diet is based solely on plant foods and restricts all animal products, including eggs and dairy.

Pros

- Since a vegan diet is plant-based, it's easier to load up on the healthy whole grains, legumes, fruits, and vegetables that many people on regular diets lack.

- Possible weight loss. If you're used to loading up on animal fats and proteins, cutting them out of your diet cuts out quite a bit of calories.

Cons

- Very limiting! Not only are animal products eliminated, but any food or product that contains an animal by-product is eliminated. No milk, butter, cheese, yogurt, or eggs.

- It can lead to possible nutrient deficiency. It's very difficult to get everything you need from plants only. In particular, vegan diets are generally lacking in calcium, protein, vitamin D, and omega-3 fatty acids.

- Difficulty dining out. If you eat at someone's home or in a restaurant, you don't have access to an ingredient list to be sure no animal products are used. For this reason, dining out can be a challenge for those who choose a vegan diet.

HCG (Human Chorionic Gonadotropin)

HCG is actually a hormone produced in the body in the earliest stages of pregnancy, which, considering how most women gain weight during that time, may seem counterintuitive to try it for weight loss. But many people have found success on this program by receiving injections and eating an extremely reduced number of calories, particularly in the beginning.

Pros

- Likely to cause rapid weight loss.

Cons

- Nutrient deficiencies often result because entire categories of foods are just blocked without any supplementation provided to make up for them.

- Safety concerns: because the calorie restriction is so low, some medical experts are concerned that HCG can set the body into starvation mode, where protein is leached from the heart, which can cause dangerous irregular contractions called ventricular tachycardia. And, if that's not bad enough for you, men who take HCG supplements or receive injections also run the risk of developing extra breast tissue.

- After reading the safety concerns, you may not be surprised to discover HCG injections are actually illegal in the US. HCG injections and supplements may only be legally marketed to treat fertility—and even then, should only be taken by prescription. However, for some reason, people show up in our clinic and talk about how they tried it and it failed for them, long term.[10]

By now you may be thinking that none of the diet plans out there are good for anybody! But, obviously, (aside from HCG) many people do find success on them. Just not everybody. If you are considering one of the above, talk to a doctor or clinic near you.

6 QUESTIONS TO ASK BEFORE STARTING ANY WEIGHT LOSS PROGRAM

1. Will I be eating REAL food?

While bars, shakes, and prepackaged foods are convenient, they rarely lead you to an empowered understanding of how to make meaningful lifestyle changes. Instead, you remain dependent on those "foods," and then when you're done with the plan, you're left to your own devices. That is the primary reason many people regain all the weight they lose on these programs soon after they go off of it.

2. Will I fix my metabolism or just lose pounds on the scale?

As Melissa's story shows, often our weight troubles arise because our metabolism is a little wonky. That means after you put in the hard work to lose weight, you risk regaining the pounds the moment you begin enjoying food again—because you didn't fix the problem.

To avoid that frustration, the program you choose should be looking at internal factors and biomarkers that influence your weight. It should be aiming to rebalance your internal environment in order to fix your metabolism, not just make you lose weight. If your metabolism improves, sustainable weight loss and weight maintenance will follow.

3. Will I see results on a meaningful timeline?

Motivation is key to losing weight, and nothing beats the scale moving downward as a powerful motivator. Many programs don't take into account that quick wins on the scale early in your journey, as well as achieving meaningful milestones afterward, are integral to staying with the program when the going gets tough.

With traditional diets, you may only lose one pound per week, which might be an OK motivator at first. But what about when you hit a plateau for three, four, five, or even six weeks? Ain't nobody got time for that!

4. Will I be held accountable, be educated, and be empowered for long-term results?

Beyond losing weight, your program should empower you to make meaningful habit changes, learn about your body, and learn about food in order to make lasting lifestyle changes. Your program should have a built-in cadence of accountability check-ins for when they matter most: AFTER you've lost weight. Accountability to keep the weight off is just as important as it is during the journey to get it off.

5. Is this customized or cookie cutter?

By now, you are well aware that cookie-cutter approaches simply don't work for everyone. They fail to take into account all the tangible and intangible factors that make a successful program work. It just doesn't make sense to even try to apply a one-size-fits-all approach to weight loss. A thirty-eight-year-old man's body is different from a post-menopausal woman's body. What makes sense is a custom plan built around your biology and your lifestyle.

6. Do you guarantee I'll see results?

If the program you're looking into won't back up their approach and assume the budget risk of you starting their program, then you may want to question if that program will really work and if it's worth the time and money to try it.

THE BEST PROGRAM GOES
BEYOND WEIGHT LOSS

It's important to find a good program so that you succeed on it! What we find so heartbreaking with many of our clients is when they give us a laundry list of diets that have failed them. We understand that weight loss is more than just about getting back into your skinny jeans. It's about your overall quality of life. And while that should be a great motivator to get started, we know it's often not enough.

If you've tried one, five, or ten times to lose weight and either failed or regained after an initial victory, it can be hard to summon the courage to try again. However, you have to keep trying because if you don't . . . well, there's no option of succeeding if you never even try. Besides, there is research that shows even if you failed numerous times, a high predictor of long-term success in weight loss is just whether you keep trying. That's right. If you keep trying, eventually you'll land on something that sticks.[11]

Doc and Dan Do: regardless of what diet or nutritional plan you are on, eat with other people whenever possible. That human connection is as good for you as proper nutrition!

There's a beautiful Spanish word frequently used in Argentina: *sobremesa*. Literally translated, it means "over table," and it refers to long meals, sometimes lasting as long as four and half hours, where people enjoy food and drink. More important, they enjoy over-the-table conversation and the strengthened relationships that result from it.

We believe one of the reasons wine has so many purported health benefits is because it is often correlated with laughing, long conversations, and spending time with loved ones in *sobremesa*.

Finding the right motivation to try yet again can be hard. Then once you start a new plan, when things get tough, it can be even harder to maintain motivation. What we've discovered in the numerous success stories from people who have come into our clinic or have worked with us from remote locations is that true, lasting motivation comes from within. If you want to lose weight to please your mate, to feel more acceptable in your social group, or to get your mother to stop hounding you, most likely you won't succeed. But if you want to lose weight for YOU—if your motivation is all about improving yourself—then you are well on your way to finding your ideal body shape.

That's why, before we get to the nitty gritty of our weight loss methods, Dan and I want to spend a few chapters discussing motivation and the psychology behind weight loss.

After you fix your metabolism, you, too, will fear no food! You'll be able to eat what you want, and whenever you gain a few pounds after you overindulged, you'll know how to get back to the weight you want to be very quickly.

But to get to that point—to follow a protocol to lose weight— requires the right mindset first.

PART II

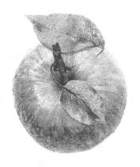

YOU GOT THIS

CHAPTER 3

GOOD HEALTH MATTERS

When Phil's wife was diagnosed with dementia, he knew what he was going to do: be right there with her, beside her, doing whatever he needed to do to take care of her. And he kept his word. He was her lone caregiver all the way to the end of her life. It was a strain physically and mentally, but he had no other choice. She was the mother of his children, the woman he promised to honor, love, and cherish until they parted in death.

After she passed away, he had a talk with his adult children. They were concerned about him because he had given everything to his wife and hadn't taken care of himself. He was stressed and overweight, and he was grieving. The kids understood, but after losing their mother, they wanted their father to be around as long as possible. So Phil promised them he'd do whatever he needed to get healthy and came to *re:vitalize* for help losing weight.

When we looked at his biodata, we discovered Phil's biological age was seventy-four—seven years older than his actual age. That didn't sit well with him. In fact, it sealed the deal. He signed on with our program that day.

Client Body Composition Biodata: Before and After Results

Phil	67 yo	6' 0"	Male			
	Before	After	Difference
Weight	243.8	185	-58.8
BMI Change/Improvement			-8
Body Fat % Lost			-11.8%
Visceral Fat Rating Improvement			-7.2
Cellular Hydration Improvement[1]			7.20%
Metabolic Improvement[2]			-38 yrs

[1] Change in body water %
[2] As measured by metabolic age reversal/improvement

Phil was eager to get through the initial stages of our nutritional approach to weight loss because he wanted his youthful metabolism back—the one where he could eat whatever he wanted. However, for the first forty days, although Phil ate a wide variety of foods, his meals were structured around what our technology discovered assimilated best with his metabolism. Our unique bioscan technology gave him a list of foods optimal for him to eat, explained how much to eat, and we went over the supplements suggested for him. It was tough on him, but not as tough as thinking he was aging faster than he wanted to be, so he stuck to it. He did so well on our program, he lost forty pounds during those first forty days.

But it wasn't just the weight loss that he was pleased with. He said his life improved on many levels. One of the first things he noticed was that it helped with his grief. Measuring out a pound of vegetables every day, checking off that he took his supplements, and drinking as much water as we told him he needed gave him something to focus on besides his grief. And in doing so, it helped him heal and find peace in his wife's passing.

In addition to that, he said his mind felt clearer now that it wasn't muddled with toxins and was being fed the nutrition it needed. But as he celebrated the numbers growing smaller on the scale, he also noticed that he was carrying himself better. His confidence was growing—he didn't feel so beaten up by life anymore. And then he realized he was so much calmer than he used to be, that stressful situations didn't bother him the way they used to.

After he shed the forty pounds, what he saw in the mirror blew him away. There was a physique that he'd forgotten he had. Feeling a little more confident because of the weight loss, he was comfortable joining a gym to improve that physique even more. Now, Phil is in such a healthier place physically and mentally that he has even begun dating again.

WEIGHT LOSS IS MORE THAN JUST PHYSICAL

Thankfully, not everyone has to deal with such emotional trauma as Phil did. But most people need to deal with the why behind their desire to lose weight just as he did. Phil's promise to his kids is what brought him into our office, but we don't believe that would have been a strong enough motivation to stick to the plan. Seeing how quickly he was aging was. It made him realize he wanted to get more out of life than he was likely going to get. And it's that internal motivation that carried him through to his end goal.

What's interesting about Phil's story is the chicken-or-the-egg metaphor that we see repeated over and over again: losing weight requires the right mindset, *but* when you lose weight, you get the right mindset to lose more or maintain it. In other words, they enable each other:

- internal motivation makes weight loss possible, and

- weight loss improves internal motivation.

So why is it so hard to tap into the right motivation to lose weight if it's always inside us? Well, that's because the reverse is also true:

- being overweight negatively impacts your self-image, and

- having a poor self-image puts you at higher risk for being overweight.

WEIGHT WALLOPS YOUR
SELF-ESTEEM

When we talk about how being overweight can really do a number to your self-esteem, we don't mean simply feeling self-conscious because you can't button your coat over your stomach. Obesity can cause clinical depression that is worsened by the tendency for self-imposed social isolation. It's tragic, but many people see their struggle with weight as a poor reflection on themselves, as if they've done something horribly wrong and are somehow less of a human being because of it.

Worsening their own poor sense of self-worth, heavy people often suffer from the treatment they receive from others. We live in an era where everyone is posting about their fabulous lives all over social media—and for some reason, no one looks overweight in those pictures! That alone can make us feel self-conscious and maybe even a bit embarrassed, but on top of that, we are often treated differently in social gatherings. Large people are shamed and deemed lazy or weak-willed to such a point that there is a stigma to being overweight. Actually, stigma isn't a strong enough word—there is a real prejudice against heavy people, as numerous studies have shown they are even paid less at work![12] Likewise, heavy children are more likely to be bullied at school, and at all ages, they tend to have a harder time making friends or dating and establishing romantic relationships.

So perhaps it only makes sense, then, that heavy folks suffer with a poor self-image. They feel unattractive and ashamed, which makes them less willing to even try to socialize. Unfortunately, that reluctance only compounds their social isolation because when they do go out, they feel awkward, and hence appear awkward. Because they are embarrassed or even feel guilty about their weight, they often avoid anything that draws attention to them. That means no sports-related activities or going places in public where others may judge them. Consequently, they frequently end up living a sedentary life, which encourages health problems due to complications from their weight.

In recent years, fat-shaming has gone under attack in many circles, but still some people justify their negative attitude toward heavy folks. They say perhaps if the overweight are shamed enough, then they will do something about their weight and health. But fat-shamers are only worsening the psychological and emotional damage heavy people have already endured.

WHY IT'S WORSE FOR
HEAVY PEOPLE

It's imperative that overweight people know they are loved unconditionally and that they get the emotional support they need. Mood disorders among heavy adolescents are common as they struggle with anger and anxiety as well as trying to hide their low self-esteem. And depression and anxiety are both common among all ages of overweight individuals. To make matters worse, remember our chicken-and-the-egg analogy? Well, there is evidence that the emotional weight heavy people carry has an impact on their physical weight and make us gain even more.[13]

Similarly, a study in *Comprehensive Psychiatry* discovered that when heavy people were able to improve their self-esteem, they were able to reverse clinical disorders, which then encouraged them to go out into public and find help for their weight.[14]

So, again, we see a cycle that can go two ways. In the first, we have low self-esteem coming from being overweight that causes depression and other emotional trauma that encourages behaviors to gain more weight, which only aggravates the feelings of low-self-esteem.

However, losing weight often gives people a psychological boost and makes them feel good about themselves. But losing is hard to do unless you're motivated to put in the work and feel good about yourself to begin with. So this cycle goes in the direction of losing weight to improve your mood, which will encourage you to lose weight.

Doc and Dan Do: spend as much time enjoying your meal as you do preparing it.

A tip we learned from our good friend Dr. Kari Anderson is to eat with mindfulness. Put your fork down between bites and focus on the full experience of eating your food by intentionally being aware of the taste, texture, and even the sounds associated with you eating.

CAN LOSING WEIGHT REALLY MAKE YOU HAPPY?

Anecdotally, Dan and I hear stories each and every day about how people's lives have changed for the better after they lose weight. They talk about how their confidence was boosted enough that they asked for (and received) pay raises, they start dating again, and they began to have more fun with the people in their lives.

Aside from the stories, though, there is plenty of evidence to back it up. In 2014, a study found that overweight people with type 2 diabetes who successfully lose weight on a program were less likely to exhibit signs of depression than those who did not lose weight.[15] And an analysis of research literature in 2011 said something similar. It found "On average, obese individuals in weight loss trials experienced reductions in symptoms of depression."[16]

Here's a fun experiment to see how easily your physiology can change your psychology.

- Raise your right arm high above your head.

- Bend your elbow to lower your hand behind your head as far as you can.

- Now, give yourself a BIG ol' pat on the back because you're awesome.

It's really hard to do this without cracking a big smile because it's a silly little exercise. But it proves that if you change your physical state, you can change how you feel.

Additionally, we've all heard about power poses too—standing tall with your arms stretched out into a victory pose, or standing like a super-hero with your chest out and hands on waist, can increase feelings of confidence.

IT'S A MATTER OF QUALITY

While we want everyone to find their internal motivation to lose weight, we cannot forget that weight loss is about improving the quality of your life. And, since our lives are built around the relationships we have with other people, that means our weight can and does impact our relationships with others. But guess what? We have yet another cycle here. Because your relationships can impact your weight, too.

For years, we've worked closely with author Dr. Kari Anderson and have shared many clients with her. In her latest book, *food, body & love*, she explains the connection between food and relationships better than anyone else we know. You can learn more about her from her website, www.myeatingdoctor.com. While that book discusses how we become vulnerable to eating disorders, her information is applicable to everyone whether they have disordered eating or not.

According to Dr. Anderson, our relationships with others are regulators of our nervous system—meaning, if we have healthy relationships, we are able to handle stress better. We're calmer, more present, and more mindful. If we do not have healthy relationships, our bodies will crave food to be our regulator. We eat to replace the quality relationships we feel we are lacking.

Before you tell yourself, "I have excellent relationships with everyone around me," take a little time to really think about your daily activities to determine if and how your weight could be interfering. Whether it's being able to easily sit on the floor (and get back up again) to play with your grandchild, the ability to run alongside your five-year-old as she learns to ride a two-wheel bike, or your willingness to be physically intimate with your partner, being overweight can discourage you from taking part in many bonding activities. Likewise, you may be less apt to join friends for a long walk on hilly terrain or an outing at the beach.

One of our clients has a collection of special automobiles that he enjoys driving and maintaining. He didn't realize his weight was interfering with that activity until he noticed he never drove his Model-A anymore and asked himself why. The answer saddened him: it was because the car was made in the early twentieth century, when people were shorter and thinner. When he sat in the car, his stomach pressed against the steering wheel and made it difficult to drive. Likewise, he wasn't getting down under his cars on the creeper seat much anymore, either, because he didn't fit as easily as he used to. He wasn't able to enjoy his hobby because of his weight.

If weight hit us all at once, it'd be easy to identify how it impacts us. But, because none of us wake up fifty pounds heavier than we were when we went to bed the night before, we kind of slide into a poorer quality of life without realizing what's happening. Maybe the realization comes when we have to buy an extender because the airplane seatbelt isn't long enough to cross our bodies. Or possibly, it's when your sister snaps at you with, "You never want to go out anymore! I'm just going to stop inviting you."

Thankfully, you don't have to hit that hard and fast realization point. We've put together a questionnaire to help you determine if your quality of life is being negatively impacted by your weight right now. Catching it early means you can tap into your internal motivation at an earlier point, too, to help encourage you on your weight loss journey.

But, even if you don't catch it early, that's okay. As Dan always says, "The best time to start was twenty years ago. The second-best time to start is today. And if not today, then start Monday (because everyone knows all good diets start on a Monday)."

Impact of Weight on Emotional Health Self-Assessment

1. Do you try to avoid getting photographed? Or stand a certain way to hide parts of your body you feel are "too much" or "embarrassing"?

2. Do you blame "old age" on your lack of activity and low energy?

3. Do you avoiding looking at yourself in the mirror?

4. When you enter a room full of people, do you look around and try to find someone who is larger than yourself and think, "Well, at least I'm not the biggest in the room"?

5. Do you find you're always adjusting your shirt around your midsection or tucking the back tail of it into your pants because it won't stay there?

6. Do you feel like you need a nap after basic activities like walking or light gardening?

7. Do you have trouble bending over to tie your shoes?

8. Do you get short of breath going up stairs?

9. Do you feel joint pain as you get moving in the morning?

10. Are your hands or feet swollen at the end of the day?

If you answered "yes" to any of the above questions, that's a sign that your weight could be negatively impacting your self-esteem, emotional health, or physical health, which means your quality of life is being negatively impacted as well.

But, let us assure you, it doesn't have to be this way. You can be happy at the weight you are—and that will actually help you lose weight. Let's look at the power of positive thinking and self-talk to help us attain the weight we want.

CHAPTER 4

POSITIVELY POSSIBLE

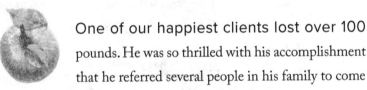 One of our happiest clients lost over 100 pounds. He was so thrilled with his accomplishment that he referred several people in his family to come see us, including Kacey, his sister-in-law. We find something special about every one of our clients, and with Kacey, we couldn't help but be impressed with her mindset! When she came in for her first consultation, she had the most beautiful positive-thinking attitude we had ever seen.

Kacey explained she was approaching her weight loss journey from a place of self-honor and self-love, instead of the self-loathing and shame many of us struggle with.

She had a ritual she'd begin with each day. She'd wake up, often still feeling exhausted as she got out of bed. As soon as she put her feet on the ground, she'd ask three questions:

- "Are you taking time to nourish yourself?"

- "Do you feel like you can keep up with your kids today?"

- "Are you ready to take on the day?"

At one point, she realized her answers had become more negative than positive. Then, one morning, she said, "No, I haven't prioritized nourishing myself in any form, through food, movement, or meditation. I am simply in self-preservation mode. I am exhausted before the day begins, and I am not looking forward to keeping up with my toddler today. I want to be a good example to my kids of someone who respects and loves herself. I want to be able to go on adventures, help them practice the sports they are learning, or play with them at a moment's notice."

Perhaps it's obvious that Kacey wasn't happy with that answer. In addition to feeling run-down personally and emotionally, she was an entrepreneur, and there were times when the tasks of growing her business just seemed to be too much. The stress was overwhelming, and she often felt as if she didn't have the reserve of energy or mental clarity she thought her work deserves.

Kacey gave herself the emotional space to breathe and contemplate what was going on. She knew she wasn't feeling as great as she wanted to and that she needed to do something about that. As she described it, she had plenty more "planned to do with this one wild and glorious life I have."

She tapped into the great love and respect she held for herself and then realized she actually led a very joyful life. And while she could honor the many talents that were uniquely hers, she knew that if she was going to be-all-and-do-all in every aspect of her life, including her health, she needed to rely on the talents and knowledge of others for a time. And she needed to get help losing weight. So that's how Kacey began her journey of caring for herself—from a place of love and kindness rather than fixing what shamed her. What a beautiful way to look at weight loss!

Ready to accept help from us, Kacey also armed herself with tools to keep her positive mindset. She said, "As I learn and become reacquainted with my body and improve my patterns so I may better care for it, I have recognized the power of mindfulness and making time for quiet. In these quiet moments of meditation come the training needed for my mind to be strong as well. The word and practice of speaking affirmations comes from the Latin word *affirmare*, meaning 'to make steady, strengthen.' That is how I choose to view my health journey: I am strengthening areas and gaining knowledge as I move toward wholeness."

And Kacey's way worked—she lost thirty-seven pounds during her first forty days on her custom *re:vitalize* weight loss plan (which is about seven pounds more than most women on our program)! We like to say she is proof positive that mindset matters.

Client Body Composition Biodata: Before and After Results

Kacey 33 yo	5' 11"	Female			
	Before	**After**	**Difference**
Weight	306.2	269.2	-37
BMI Change/Improvement			-5.2
Body Fat % Lost			-12.0%
Visceral Fat Rating Improvement			-2.4
Cellular Hydration Improvement[1]			+3.1%
Metabolic Improvement[2]			-37 yrs

[1] Change in body water %
[2] As measured by metabolic age reversal/improvement

WATCH HOW YOU TALK
ABOUT YOURSELF

Few of us realize the extent to which we speak to ourselves in a negative way. That's because we don't ever step on a scale and directly say, "Self, you are not acceptable." But we do step on a scale and interpret our emotions—which is one of the ways we do talk to ourselves. If we feel despair or shame, we're telling ourselves we did something wrong. Unfortunately, people are not motivated by shame—embarrassment makes us want to hide or, worse, sneak food and eat to try to feel better.

Doc and Dan Do: eat like you give a damn about yourself! This is a concept we learned from Dr. Anderson. It's about making choices from the perspective of who you want to be or of someone you esteem. Whom do you admire? A star athlete? Then ask yourself, "Would a star athlete choose to fuel themselves this way?" How do you want to live? As a vibrant and energetic person? Then ask yourself, "Would a vibrant and energetic person choose to fuel themselves this way?" If the answer is "no," then think twice before that indulgence. It doesn't mean you can't or shouldn't indulge, but do so with the right mindset.

Of course, another way we talk to ourselves *does* involve words: the words we use in our thoughts as well as the ones that come out of our mouths. Kacey's story is a powerful example of what it looks like to choose the right words. Instead of letting her feelings of shame or anger or any other negative emotion keep her in an unmotivated state of despair, she came to her weight loss goal from a place of acknowledging that she mattered, that she was a valuable and loved human being, that she had gifts yet to give, and if she was going to give them, she needed to take charge of her health.

Feeling empowered, she made the choices that set her on a trajectory to become healthier and lose the weight. Kacey shows us that sometimes the hardest work you need to do in order to attain your weight goals may just take place between your ears.

Perhaps nothing demonstrates the power of your mind on your weight better than a 2013 study done by researchers in the Netherlands of women with anorexia.[17] These women had repeated thoughts that told themselves they were "too big" or "too fat" so frequently that they believed it to the point where they couldn't actually see themselves correctly. The women were observed walking through doorways. As they walked through, they would turn their shoulders as if they needed to squeeze sideways to fit, although there was plenty of room for them.

It's amazing to think about it, but their brains had repeated the "I'm too big" self-talk so much that it was unable to interpret the world through any other filter! As they worked on improving self-talk, their image adjusted, and eventually they were able to walk through the doorway facing forward.

This study demonstrates that our beliefs about ourselves impact the way we interpret and experience the world. But beliefs can change; after all, a belief is just a repeated thought. If you frequently engage in negative self-talk about yourself, you'll develop beliefs that, in turn, will alter your perception and encourage behaviors and choices that can fit exactly what that negative self-talk says. And, if you do the opposite, and repeat positive thoughts about yourself, your beliefs will change to reflect those thoughts.

Dan actually experienced this very phenomenon while writing this book. Although he was very athletic, he really didn't enjoy cardio or running. To put it the way he did, he "haaaaaaaaaaaated" running or any other kind of cardiovascular exercise that didn't involve chasing a ball.

When his gym was forced to close due to the COVID-19 pandemic, he needed to find an alternative form of exercise. A friend wanted him to run with him, so he did, reluctantly and not expecting any kind of love affair with the activity. One day, after he returned home from a run, he thought he'd (once again) tell his wife how much he haaaaaaaaaaated running, how he couldn't stand to do any cardio, how he—but his wife wanted a change of topic.

"Let me interrupt you, real quick," Danae said. "Think about it. If you keep telling yourself and everyone else that you 'hate cardio' or that 'cardio is the worst,' you're never going to enjoy it. You need to change your language if you're ever going to learn to tolerate it, let alone love doing it."

Dan's a wise man. He knows to listen to his wife. So he worked on how he spoke about running. And now he's running over thirty miles a week and genuinely loving it. In fact, he just completed a marathon.

Observe how you talk about and to yourself. If you repeatedly say, "I hate vegetables," what kind of foods do you think you'll choose from a restaurant menu? The steamed vegetable for a side or the French fries? If you associate yourself with a particular image, what do you think you will look like? Something we hear way too often in our clinic, especially among the men, is "guys like me will always be big." What they don't realize they're saying is "guys who talk this way to themselves this way will always be big."

To help improve self-talk, we encourage all our clients to take the time to incorporate positive affirmations into their daily routine. You may be familiar with positive affirmations, or at least have seen greeting cards or memes of SNL's Stuart Smalley character that end with "and goshdarnit, people like me!" But if you're not familiar with them, positive affirmations are short, motivating, or inspiring statements you repeat out loud to yourself.

The repetition is important because, basically, what you're doing is training your brain to get in the habit of thinking kind thoughts about yourself and feeling the positive emotions that accompany it. Because here's the kicker: when you repeat a thought over and over and over, your brain makes it part of your belief system. That's why if you habitually tell yourself you can't eat any cake because you can never stop at just one bite, then you'll prove yourself right. However, if you repeatedly tell yourself that you are always able to control yourself with all foods, then you will prove yourself right that way, too.

Because we encourage people to say them out loud, they often balk at the idea. And we get it. It does feel kind of silly when you first start doing them, as if you're engaging in some kind of woo-woo activity. But if you rely on repeating them silently to yourself, it's easier to get distracted.

Another thing that makes doing affirmations a little tricky is that you have to choose what you say very carefully. If you force yourself to say something that you consciously reject over and over, you will probably never see the results you want. For as much mental effort as you put into saying them, you'll be putting equal effort into rejecting them. You will feel as if you're wasting your time and will become frustrated with the whole practice.

So instead of trying to repeat, "I always fill myself up with vegetables at every meal," while you're thinking about how much you hate vegetables, think of something you can believe. "I like to take care of myself. I feel good when I make healthy choices." Those kinds of statements are easier for most of us to believe. And repeating them will encourage you to make better choices when it comes to feeding yourself.

Another way of choosing good affirmations and of training your brain to talk nicely to yourself is to think about how an ideal parent would speak to you. We got this idea from Dr. Anderson and absolutely love it.

POSITIVE PARENTING

T hink about how an ideal parent speaks to their child. They say statements that come from the heart, from an authentic place of care. Would such a parent ever tell their three-year-old "you're fat and lazy"? No! They would have compassion, patience, understanding, and love. They would not be critical. They would never see that child as a failure. They would realize the three-year-old is a perfectly imperfect human being—as we all are—who is trying to do the best it can. And that the child's best is good enough.

Compare that ideal parent's way of communicating with the way you communicate with yourself. Do you frequently tell yourself encouraging or comforting words? Or do you often remind yourself of your flaws? Do you congratulate yourself for all your wins, regardless of how small? Or do you complain about what you didn't do correctly and fret over it?

Being an ideal parent to yourself requires you remain vigilant in your thoughts to catch yourself in the act of being unkind to yourself so you can course-correct. Making new positive patterns of thought about yourself will probably be one of the hardest things you ever decide to do—but it's also one of the most important things you can do. So, to make it easier for people, one of the tools Dr. Anderson uses to help her patients learn to speak to themselves in this way is to have them do a journaling exercise. She asks them to spend time each day writing letters to themselves from the perspective of the perfect parent.

Granted, for some, pretending to be the perfect parent to themselves might be a bit too touchy-feely. For those folks, finding a new strategy to talk to and about yourself might require thinking about your identity and what you identify as.

IDENTIFYING YOUR AWESOME SELF

When Danae challenged Dan to change the way he speaks to himself about running, she was really asking him to change the way he identified himself. For years, Dan had told himself he was not a runner, not only that, but he was the kind of person who hated running and found little value in doing cardio.

When he took her advice, he had to figure out a way to change how he spoke about running. He couldn't just outright say "I love running" (yet). He rejected that idea so vehemently that he couldn't take himself seriously. Instead, he tried to change his identity to one of being a runner. He asked, "How does a runner think and feel about himself?" and tried to create some positive affirmations from that. He figured a runner:

- enjoyed feeling strong,

- enjoyed feeling accomplished, and

- felt at ease with his body's movements.

So, when he'd think about running, he'd stop to breathe and say a few affirmations based on what he thought a runner felt:

I enjoy feeling strong. I love feeling accomplished. I like it when I feel at ease with my body's movement.

Those statements motivated him somewhat, so he expanded and came up with some statements he could believe that were about running:

- I like the idea of running.

- I like how good I feel after a run.

- I like how mindful I am when I run.

You might be able to guess, soon he was saying, "I love to run" and meant it.

Try changing your identity a little and ask what that new person thinks and feels. Don't wait until after you lose weight before you tell yourself, "I'm a healthy person." Ask how does a healthy person walk, act, eat? And most importantly, how do healthy people talk to themselves?

The key to positive affirmations working for you is that you feel good when you say them. You might have to start in a somewhat abstract or general place. With the example of identifying as a healthy person, that might be hard to do after leaving the doctor's office and being lectured about your lab results. In that case, think about other habits that a healthy person may engage in. You might find your starting point is something like:

A healthy person wears comfortable clothing. I like comfortable clothing. I wear comfortable clothing because that's what a healthy person wears.

Regardless of where you start changing your thoughts and self-talk, if you do so with the intention of always reaching for more positive expressions, you will find yourself thinking more positively about yourself when you're not doing positive affirmations. They kind of get the ball rolling in the right direction for you. When you do feel good about yourself, keep it up. Positive affirmations require regular practice! It's too easy to slide back into negative thinking, especially in today's era of non-stop media and social sharing.

REALLY? POSITIVE AFFIRMATIONS WORK?

We get it. Sometimes you feel silly saying positive affirmations out loud. So, if you need some convincing that they really do work to change the way you think, feel, and act in the world, here are some compelling studies to back them up:

- In 1988, Claude M. Steele, now a professor emeritus at Stanford, looked at the power of self-affirmational responses among people dealing with addictive behaviors. In particular, he wondered whether taking a moment to stop and affirm a value that was important to self-concept would help a person resist indulging in their addiction. He discovered such self-talk did, indeed, help.[18] The people who engaged in self-affirmational practices chose to abstain from their addictive behaviors when given the opportunity to indulge. Dr. Steele later went on to demonstrate how self-affirmation encouraged better attitudes and healthy behaviors[19] in general.

- In 2015, a study found that, if used consistently, not only do positive affirmations promote healthy behaviors, but they make us more resilient. When faced with a negative remark or something that threatens our sense of self-worth, positive affirmations help people remain secure in their identity and remain feeling competent.[20]

- And finally, there's a pretty amazing study that involves 326 cancer survivors. It proves the power of positive thoughts can actually impact physical health by concluding that people who were optimistic wound up having better health outcomes.[21]

Hopefully by now you're convinced that thinking positively and speaking positively about yourself is something you need to attain your weight loss goals. If you need help getting started, here are some generalized ones that you can use until you build enough momentum that you come up with some of your own. Remember, though, you need to believe yourself as you say them, so if one of these feels off, skip it and go on to the next. (For ideas on positive affirmations, check out our appendix for some awesome ones to get started with.)

Although we introduced the concept of positive self-talk as a way to help get you started on your weight loss journey, please know you need to keep the talk going. As with any large change in your life, you will go through several stages. Each will have its own challenges and benefits, and the way you talk to yourself will definitely help you flip the balance of those so that you experience more benefits than challenges.

IT'S GOOD FOR YOUR HEALTH

You probably get it by now: losing weight is a great way to improve the quality of your life, and the only way you'll find lasting motivation to stick to a weight loss plan is by taking control of your mind. It has to be *your* decision, and then *you* have to be the one to stick to that decision. But one thing we haven't really spoken about to this point is how losing weight can impact your physical health as well as your mental health. So, for a little more motivation to get your thoughts aligned with losing weight, let's talk a little bit about the connection between your weight and your health.

CHAPTER 5

IT'S NOT
JUST A MATTER
OF POUNDS

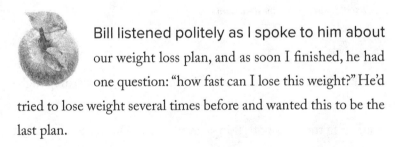 Bill listened politely as I spoke to him about our weight loss plan, and as soon I finished, he had one question: "how fast can I lose this weight?" He'd tried to lose weight several times before and wanted this to be the last plan.

What was most important to Bill was lowering his BMI, drastically. In fact, he was obsessed with it. BMI stands for Body Mass Index. It is a height-to-weight metric used by medical professionals, insurance companies, and the CDC to give general guidance on how much a person *should* weigh given their height. We tend to be critical of this metric as a sole predictor of health because it doesn't take into account things like muscle mass or bone density, but as you'll see with Bill's story, some surgeons use it as a way to mitigate certain risks in surgery.

Client Body Composition Biodata: Before and After Results

Bill 71 yo | 6' 1" | Male			
	Before	**After**	**Difference**
Weight	377.2	334.2	-43
BMI Change/Improvement			-5.7
Body Fat % Lost			-29.4%
Visceral Fat Rating Improvement			-22

See, Bill was a busy and successful man. He had a rewarding high-level corporate job, and he sidelined as a popular entertainer and marketing trainer—both things he considered his passion projects. Unfortunately, he had to retire from both those passions because of what he thought was back pain and a "pinched" nerve, or nerve impingement, all caused by arthritis.

However, after several consultations, X-rays, MRIs, and even a few outpatient surgeries, it was discovered that Bill's hip joint was the real issue. Yes, he had arthritis, and that had completely fused the parts of his hip, rendering it useless. Not only that, but the fusion impacted the nerve that ran from his lower spine to his knee in such a way that it became the actual cause of the vast majority of his pain.

As soon as he learned his hip was the true cause, he started looking for a surgeon to replace it. He and his wife began to research clinics and surgeons, thinking it would be an easy thing to do. After all, it seemed as if every other person over a certain age had had a hip replacement. But they soon discovered it wouldn't be easy for him to join their ranks. In fact, that's when all hopes of ever being normal again seemed to be dashed.

See, Bill knew he was heavy, but according to the doctors, he was "morbidly obese." That meant he wasn't even close to being a candidate for hip replacement surgery because a high BMI could lead to the body not "accepting" the artificial joint being implanted. He'd tried with four different orthopedic clinics and received the same responses: if he could substantially reduce his BMI, they'd do the surgery.

Bill's life went on hold as he tried diet after diet to lose weight, all to no avail. Meanwhile, both his pain and lack of mobility increased—until Bill heard an advertisement on the radio for our clinic.

When he went on our program, he literally shrank. Several months later, he returned to his first choice to do the hip replacement surgery.

His doctor ran a bunch of tests and greeted him with, "You need a new hip! Let's get it scheduled." There was no mention about BMI or weight loss; instead, he insisted Bill get the surgery right away—something Bill agreed with whole-heartedly.

YOUR HEALTH AND YOUR WEIGHT

As Bill's story shows us, being overweight can interfere with other needs, like surgery. But several health complications are actually caused by being overweight. Overweight people are at higher risk of developing cardiovascular diseases, atherosclerosis, diabetes, and high blood pressure. And being overweight puts you at higher risk for developing certain types of cancer, osteoarthritis, and back pain.[22]

The good news is, by losing weight, you can lower your risks for all those conditions and even reverse certain ones. Just dropping 5 to 10 percent of your body weight will lower your cholesterol, improve your blood pressure, and lower your blood sugar levels.[23]

Even better, you can completely reverse some conditions by losing weight! Research out of Washington University found that when obese people lost weight, they also reversed "significant heart health problems."[24] Bad cholesterol drops, good cholesterol rises, and tri-glycerides lower, too, when there is less fat on a person's body. All that means the chance of you having a heart attack or stroke decreases when you lose weight. In addition to that, you can decrease your body's inflammation. The fat cells in your belly actually encourage inflammation by releasing certain chemicals that are irritants to your body's tissues. This inflammation is a contributor to heart disease, stroke, and arthritis.[25]

Many people who lose weight through a healthy diet are able to go off their medications for type 2 diabetes and still maintain healthy blood sugar levels.[26] Anecdotally, we find in our clinics that, on any given month, between 20 to 40 percent of our clients are coming off of or reducing their obesity-related medications according to a self-reported survey. Folks with sleep apnea are able to get a better night's sleep, and some can even go off their CPAP machines when they lose weight.[27] And here's something really hopeful: when overweight women are able to lose 5 percent of their body weight, they cut their odds of getting breast cancer by 12 percent![28]

It's unfortunate and even sad, but every day more and more Americans wind up taking medications for this condition or that condition. Yes, some medications are required to help certain people manage their health, but many folks wind up with a medicine cabinet full of pharmaceuticals with harmful side effects that only address the symptoms they are experiencing. Those pills do not fix the underlying cause. And we have seen time and time again that when our patients lose weight, they can eliminate most if not all their medications.

BUT WAIT! THERE'S MORE!

You don't have to have a diagnosed medical condition in order to benefit from losing weight. Your body will feel better, and you'll have more energy as well. Think about some of these statistics:

- Every ten extra pounds of weight on your body adds forty pounds of pressure on your knees and ankles! That extra wear and tear can lead to pain, stiffness, and arthritis.

- Your sleep improves! We already mentioned how sleep apnea improves with weight loss, but many overweight people suffer insomnia and have trouble sleeping all night. It's believed that obesity somehow changes a person's metabolism in such a way that it messes up their regular sleep cycle rhythms.[29]

- We touched on this already, but it's so important that it's worth repeating: losing weight can lift your mood! Researchers have actually found that overweight depressed people who lose at least 8 percent of their bodyweight are happier after the weight loss.[30]

- Improved sex life! Heavier folks report being less comfortable being intimate with their partners, and even if they are comfortable, there is a link between being overweight and having less desire.[31]

As you can see, being overweight or obese can be a significant detriment to your overall health. And we noticed that much of the research for the above statistics mentioned that the improvements were discovered at a weight loss of only about 5 or 10 percent of your body weight. You may not need to lose much weight at all in order to feel significantly better.

If you're still on the fence about whether losing weight is worth the effort, there's one more stat we'd like to introduce to you. It's one our client Evan learned from his cardiologist. After his uncle had passed away from a heart attack at only fifty years old, Evan thought he'd get checked out by a cardiologist. He was in his thirties at the time, with a young son and a wife pregnant with his daughter. The day he got his lab results, the doctor wanted to know some important information:

"Do you want to walk your daughter down the aisle when she gets married," he asked, "or do you want some other guy to do it?"

Of course, Evan wanted to be there. But his doctor assured him unless he lost some weight, he may never see the day. That's right: being overweight can lead to an early demise. For people who qualify as severely obese, a BMI of forty or more, their life expectancy can be reduced by as much as twenty years!

Client Body Composition Biodata:
Before and After Results

Evan	47 yo | 5' 11" | Male		
	Before	**After**	**Difference**
Weight	259.2	230.2	-29
BMI Change/Improvement			-4.1
Body Fat % Lost			-9.1%
Visceral Fat Rating Improvement			-5.9
Cellular Hydration Improvement[1]			+4.2%
Metabolic Improvement[2]			-34 yrs

[1] Change in body water %
[2] As measured by metabolic age reversal/improvement

WHAT'S THE DEAL WITH
THE BMI?

A person's BMI can indicate how much of their body is made of excess fat. According to the Centers for Disease Control (CDC):

- If your BMI is less than 18.5, you are underweight.

- If your BMI is 18.5 to <25, you are of normal weight.

- If your BMI is 25.0 to <30, you are overweight.

- If your BMI is 30.0 or higher, you are considered obese.[32]

People who register as obese are at risk for a host of medical complications, including an increased risk of hospital readmission after hip surgery, additional operations, infections, artificial joint infection, and sepsis (a life-threatening infection).[33] And yet obesity isn't rare. In 2017–2018, 42.4 percent of the US population were considered obese.[34]

Are you wondering what your BMI is? You can do a little math to determine the ratio of your weight to your height and find out. Take your weight in kilograms and divide it by the square of your height in meters.

THE BMI IS
NOT FOOLPROOF

Although the medical community relies on the BMI as an indicator of whether someone is at a healthy weight, it does have its critics. As mentioned earlier, we don't put that much stock in the BMI as a good metric tool. Seriously, if you took the BMI of competitive bodybuilders, you would discover they are considered obese! And, as reported in the *Wall Street Journal*, one of the troubles with the BMI is that it treats people as two-dimensional; it suggests that as we get taller, we should get wider.[35] Thankfully, that's not the case. Another problem with it is that it doesn't take into consideration that men and women have different types of bodies.

Still, it's agreed that we need a baseline for what a healthy weight is to determine, in part, what range puts someone at risk for health conditions related to being overweight. So, to get a better idea of whether a person is at a good weight for them, we take their body frame into consideration, as well as looking at their BMI. Our biometric technology is one of our most reliable tools to do this as it shows a more holistic picture of a person's health. It looks at body-fat percentage, hydration level, visceral fat ratings, muscle mass, and even metabolic age.

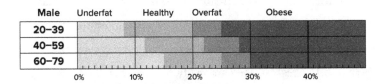

Female	Underfat	Healthy	Overfat	Obese
20–39				
40–59				
60–79				

0%   10%   20%   30%   40%

Male	Underfat	Healthy	Overfat	Obese
20–39				
40–59				
60–79				

0%   10%   20%   30%   40%

Desirable Ranges:

Everybody needs fat. The chart above depicts the various ranges of fat with respect to age and sex. Research has shown that individuals with appropriate amounts of fat are less likely to develop obesity-related health conditions.

Body Fat % Goal:

Body fat % is a much more accurate indication of your weight-related status than BMI, which is essentially a height and weight chart.

The *re:vitalize Program* is designed to target abnormal fat.

Set a realistic goal for your body fat % and then follow the plan. While on the re:vitalize program the goal is not just to lose weight but to lose body fat and body fat % and gain body water %. When everything is going in the right direction, this will lower your metabolic age (increasing your metabolism). It is a great goal to have your metabolic age substantially lower than your actual age.

In addition, we suggest our clients use biometric body composition scales that are now on the market. They use a technology called "electric impedance" and sync up to your smart phone to give you all sorts of biodata, then communicate via Bluetooth to your phone to give you data on your weight, BMI, body fat percentage, fat-free body weight, subcutaneous fat (the kind under your skin), visceral fat (the very unhealthy kind that surrounds your organs), body hydration level, metabolic age, and so much more. We periodically review new scales on the market. See our recommendations by signing up for the free resources accompanying this book at fearnofoodbook.com.

Keep in mind, no measurements or measuring devices will always be perfect for everybody. You may have some numbers that seem out of range, but because of your bone structure, your exercise level, or some other reason, they are really only artificially out of range.

WHAT'S A GOOD WEIGHT FOR ME?

We believe it only makes sense that people who are "bigger boned" should weigh more than their counterparts with smaller frames. So we use something called the "wrist method" to determine a person's frame, then match their height with a weight to determine whether they should lose weight to improve their health and by how much. We also have two charts to make that determination: one for women and one for men. The wrist method works like this:

- Wrap your thumb and second finger around your wrist.

    ✓ If your fingers overlap, you have a small body frame.

    ✓ If your fingers touch, then you have a medium body frame.

✓ If there is a gap between your fingers, then you have a large body frame.

Now that you know what kind of frame you have, use the following charts to determine if you are within a healthy body weight. The weight ranges are in pounds.

How Much Weight Do You Need to Lose?

Use the simple "wrist method" for a general idea of how much weight you need to lose. Here's how it works: wrap your wrist using your thumb and second finger.

If your fingers overlap:	If your fingers touch:	If your fingers don't touch:
Small Body Frame	**Medium Body Frame**	**Large Body Frame**

SUGGESTED WEIGHT CHART FOR MEN

HEIGHT	Small Frame	Medium Frame	Large Frame
5'2"	128-134	131-141	138-150
5'3"	130-136	133-143	140-153
5'4"	132-138	135-145	142-156
5'5"	134-140	137-148	144-160
5'6"	136-142	139-151	146-164
5'7"	138-145	142-154	149-168
5'8"	140-148	145-157	152-172
5'9"	142-151	148-160	155-176
5'10"	144-154	151-163	158-180
5'11"	146-157	154-166	161-184
6'0"	149-160	157-170	164-188
6'1"	152-164	160-174	168-192
6'2"	155-168	164-178	172-197
6'3"	158-172	167-182	176-202
6'4"	162-176	171-187	181-207

SUGGESTED WEIGHT CHART FOR WOMEN

HEIGHT	Small Frame	Medium Frame	Large Frame
4'10"	102-111	109-121	118-131
4'11"	103-113	111-123	120-134
5'0"	104-115	113-126	122-137
5'1"	106-118	115-129	125-140
5'2"	108-121	118-132	128-143
5'3"	111-124	121-135	131-147
5'4"	114-127	124-138	134-151
5'5"	117-130	127-141	137-155
5'6"	120-133	130-144	140-159
5'7"	123-136	133-147	143-163
5'8"	126-139	136-150	146-167
5'9"	129-142	139-153	149-170
5'10"	132-145	142-156	152-173
5'11"	135-148	145-159	155-176
6'0"	138-151	148-162	158-179

WHERE IS THE PLAN?

B y now, you know why it's so easy to gain weight and why different people need different plans to help them lose weight. You also understand that the first step to losing weight is getting control of your thoughts to find your internal motivation, then retraining your brain to think more positively about your ability to lose the weight. You also understand the true impact of weight on your health.

If, after looking at the BMI and wrist-method charts, you think you need to lose some weight, the next section is probably what you've been waiting for: our nutritional plan, which helps you shed the pounds and fix your metabolism and finally *fear no food*.

PART III

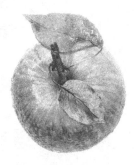

HERE'S WHAT WORKS

CHAPTER 6

HOW TO BE
A LOSER

Pastor Steve has a big heart, and he serves a big congregation. And after years of several meetings a week in coffee shops and diners, he developed a big physique, too. At least, one that was bigger than he wanted it to be.

With a family history of high blood pressure and cholesterol problems, Pastor Steve was concerned that, in addition to the weight slowing down his busy life, it was putting him at risk for health conditions. Then, because doctors are good at pointing out what's wrong with us, Pastor Steve's doctor confirmed that, yes, he needed to lose some weight, and prescribed him medication for cholesterol. However, the doctor did say if he could lose a little weight, that would go a long way toward helping his big heart stay healthy.

So Pastor Steve began jogging. When he was younger, jogging had helped maintain his weight. But as happens with many of us who have to scroll a little further to click our age on online drop-down menus, jogging either wasn't working or was not working as quickly as it used to. That number on the scale just wasn't budging. But he doubled down on the exercise and started reviewing diets.

Unfortunately, as he was beginning to struggle in earnest to lose the weight, Pastor Steve received some bad news. His father had been diagnosed with a quickly progressing cancer and was given fewer than two months to live. Pastor Steve forgot about the need to diet, and instead shifted his focus to ensure his father had the best quality of life possible for as long as he could.

His father beat the odds and actually lived another two years. That whole time, Pastor Steve was at the ready for whatever Dad needed—taking him to appointments, ensuring his medications were right, keeping him company, and making him know how loved and appreciated he was. But after his father passed away, Pastor Steve realized he hadn't been taking care of himself much at all. And when he stepped on a scale, he saw a number he'd never expected. All that comfort eating had put him in an uncomfortable position. A very unhealthy one, too.

Being realistic about his lifestyle, he recognized he'd need to figure out how to lose the weight in a way that was in alignment with his schedule and with his frequent in-restaurant meals. He wanted a program with real food that he could use in real life. And that's what he found with the *re:vitalize weight loss* program. He lost forty pounds, and two years later, he still can't find it. He'd like to lose a little more, but his wife disagrees, saying something about how hard it was to find him behind the pulpit.

The best part of the weight loss for Pastor Steve is that his lifestyle hasn't changed too drastically. He loves food and still gets to eat whatever he wants (even unhealthy fare in moderation). He can travel, have numerous meetings in restaurants each week, and still maintain his weight.

As with many of us, Pastor Steve's favorite moments and special family gatherings are celebrated with food. Times of bonding, sharing, and joy are only made better and often commemorated with traditional meals. Pastor Steve didn't want to give that up. But he also knows that overdoing it will put a tight limit on how many of those events he'd be able to show up to if his life were cut short. As he says, genetics are the bullets you're given; how you use them in the gun is your lifestyle. He has chosen to use his bullets with the intention of enjoying life's pleasures without damaging his health.

Without the excess weight holding him back, his energy level has skyrocketed and he's sleeping much better than before. He attributes that sleep to his optimistic outlook on life. It's hard to feel hopeful when you're exhausted, and so much easier to live in hope and positivity when you're rested and energized.

Pastor Steve believes that losing weight and beginning to feel better affects people internally—it affects their soul, their spirit. As he says, we are primarily a spirit with a body. There's integration between the two, and when our body's not in a good place, it affects our spirit as well.

SO WHAT WORKS?

Pastor Steve, as with the others we've mentioned in this book, found success on our program because he followed it to a T. What does that mean? Because we have a custom-tailored approach for everybody, it's never exactly the same. But there are a few things we've found that work among our thousands of clients regardless of age, gender, underlying medical conditions, etc. We consider them pillars for any effective weight loss plan. However, don't stress about the need to immediately adopt each one right now. Treat these different ideas as you would a buffet—experiment with a few for a couple days or weeks. Once you feel confident with them, incorporate another, then another when you feel ready.

Here's a rundown of what we know helps just about everyone lose weight.

Intermittent Fasting

We encourage all our clients to "do" intermittent fasting. What that means is that you choose a targeted time of the day for all of your eating. We call it your "eating window." There are many different methods and much research out there on how and why to take advantage of intermittent fasting. But, if it's your first time trying this out, we suggest an eight-hour period for eating. Maybe it's from eleven o'clock in the morning to seven o'clock in the evening. Or noon to eight in the evening. Whatever eight-hour window is most convenient for you, that's when you'll eat. The other sixteen hours of your day should only include water or indulging in zero-calorie drinks.

Although you can choose any eating window you want, most folks find it easiest to start their fast after dinner (the night before), go to sleep without snacks, skip breakfast the next morning, then proceed to eat their first meal the following day around lunch time. Throughout the day, you may eat as often as you'd like as long as your last meal is before your eight hours end. For the rest of the day and the next morning before you start eating again, we recommend hot tea, black coffee, or sugar-free carbonated beverages that can blunt cravings or hunger pangs.

Intermittent fasting is a simple, regulated way to eat, but it's also a very healthy thing to do. There are numerous benefits realized from adapting an intermittent fasting lifestyle. The one that most people like to hear about it is that it promotes weight loss by requiring the body to burn off fat stores as fuel. It also regulates blood sugar levels, which prevents spikes and crashes. And it allows your digestive system an opportunity to rest and recover.

Isn't breakfast the most important meal of the day? That's probably the question we receive the most frequently when we first introduce intermittent fasting. And yeah, marketers working for cereal companies over the past fifty years sure have made it look that way. But science doesn't back that up.[36] Sure, some people love breakfast and they do well on it, but not everybody. And there are plenty of health benefits from skipping breakfast.

> Doc and Dan Do: skip breakfast three to four days each week and then try to do a full day fast (dinner to dinner) at least once a month.

Probably the best part of intermittent fasting is that it has some very beneficial side effects. One is it lowers your insulin levels and may help prevent type 2 diabetes.[37] But that is just the tip of the iceberg. Intermittent fasting improves biometric markers (we'll discuss those further in Chapter 8), which basically means it helps us age slower. It reduces oxidative stress—the stuff that makes us prone to illnesses. It improves cognition, meaning we think more clearly, and it has an anti-inflammatory effect.[38] And, anecdotally, many of our clients claim that allowing their digestive systems to rest just a couple extra hours at night has had significant digestive benefits. Since their bodies were not perpetually overfed, their digestive systems didn't have to work so hard to break down their food.

Aside from all that, intermittent fasting is considered one of the most natural ways of eating. Let's face it, our early ancestors didn't get out of bed, go downstairs, and pour a cup of coffee from their programmed coffee pot and pull something out of the fridge to nuke and eat. They woke up, stretched, maybe scratched an itch, then wandered outside to look for a berry or two to eat for brunch. At the end of the day, they were back home snuggling around the fire with nothing sweet or salty or crunchy to snack on before bed. In other words, they were intermittent fasters.

But while all that might be interesting to you, you're reading this book for weight loss help. And the good news here is that there is evidence intermittent fasting helps you actively lose weight. The hormone adiponectin, which helps the brain increase energy expenditure (burn more calories), increases in people who do intermittent fasting.[39]

Pretty amazing, eh? And all you have to do is eat within an eight-hour window!

But there are caveats! If you suffer from low blood sugar or diabetes, utilizing intermittent fasting may require you to be more mindful of your blood sugar regulation. In these cases, we ask that you break your eating window up a little and have pure protein in the mornings—like two hard-boiled eggs or a small serving of lean meat. And as always, consult your doctor before taking this approach, particularly if you have blood sugar issues.

And one final word about intermittent fasting: don't feel like you need to use this protocol every single day of your life. You can still achieve many of the benefits of intermittent fasting even if you're only following it a few days per week.

Hydrate

Because all of our metabolic processes start and end in the cell, perhaps it only makes sense to look at the cellular level to see what we can do to ensure our cells are putting out optimum performance. And that brings us to the second, and arguably most important, element of our weight loss protocol: ensuring you are getting adequate hydration at the cellular level. When your cells are dehydrated, they cannot function well, and that means a lot of processes related to weight loss are inhibited. Your liver's ability to metabolize fat is weakened. Your growth hormone, which is needed to break down fat cells, is reduced. Lipase is also reduced; that is an enzyme that's needed to metabolize fat. And our cognitive function declines, which makes us feel tired. You know what happens when we feel tired? We crave carbs as a source of quick fuel.[40]

Perhaps now you see why many crash diets that cause you to lose a lot of water weight cannot give you long-term weight loss results. Your cells just can't function and metabolize anything if they are shrunken up with dehydration. So then you yo-yo and gain back the weight (sometimes more) the moment you daydream about a donut. Therefore, we need to ensure your cells are properly hydrated so they can do what they're designed to do.

But proper hydration, particularly cellular hydration, goes beyond just making sure you're drinking enough water. It's a function of quantity (are you getting enough water) and quality (does the water have the right trace minerals or electrolytes to make it usable once it's in your body).

As for quantity, everyone's body is different. A general rule of thumb is to aim for drinking half your body weight in ounces of water each day. If you weigh 200 pounds, you should drink 100 ounces of water each day.

As for quality . . . we've all heard of electrolytes, right? Gatorade has made those a household name for many of us. An electrolyte is simply a trace mineral that creates a slight electrical charge on the cell membrane, which draws water molecules into the cell. If our bodies don't have the right trace mineral balance (lack of quality), we may be drinking plenty of water (quantity), but our body isn't absorbing that hydration at the cellular level. We're either just peeing it straight out, or it "pools" as puffy interstitial fluid (unhelpful water outside the cells) in our ankles or wrists.

See, much of the water we drink is purified or distilled in some way to remove harmful contaminants and chemicals. We're all for removing those things, *but*, in that process, the trace minerals and electrolytes our cells need to function properly are also removed. In other words, we can drink a ton of water each day and not actually get the proper hydration we need at the cellular levels. That explains why so many of our clients, who have assured us they are properly hydrated when we first see them in the office, are shocked to discover when we take their biodata that they really are dehydrated. They've been drinking a lot of water, just not the right water.

One way to ensure proper hydration for your cells is by supplementing with a high-quality trace mineral supplement. That will feed your cells the electrolytes and other minerals it needs so it will relax, open up, and allow the water to go through it. And here's the good news: it's incredibly easy to find the trace minerals you need. They are in pink salt! I'll spare you the biology lesson here, but water needs help finding the way into your cells, and pink salt, unlike typical table salt, is a great source of electrolytes—the minerals that help hydrate you.

Too much salt in any form is bad for you. But, if you eat a very healthy diet primarily of vegetables and fruits, then you may be at risk of not getting enough sodium. Instead of reaching for the white, refined table salt, we encourage the use of high-quality pink salt. It's not refined and has magnesium and other important minerals you need to nourish your cells and allow for proper hydration.

If you give up all processed foods (no breads, pastas, premade convenience foods, etc.) then you may need to add salt to your diet to get your daily minimum requirement of sodium. We encourage pink salt because it has the minerals and electrolytes (like magnesium) that your body will crave to hydrate it.

Avoid Added Sugar

Once you develop the habit of reading food labels to look for sugars, you'll be shocked at how much sugar is hidden in just about everything! Our most successful clients learn to identify these added sugars and then opt for alternatives. But we're not here to demonize sugar entirely. Sugar occurs naturally in all foods that contain carbohydrates (including fruits, veggies, and grains), which tells us that not all sugar is bad for us. However, whole foods that give us sugar also provide us with essential minerals, antioxidants, and fiber. These foods are slowly digested, so they give us good nutrition *and* provide our bodies with a steady source of energy. On the other hand, refined white sugar and its other buddies (like high fructose corn syrup) give us a massive dump of energy that we can't possibly use up easily, so it quickly goes to fat storage without any of the nutrition.

So we need to be mindful about sugar, particularly when it is *added* sugar that food manufacturers use to extend shelf life and increase flavor. We don't need to warn you about the obvious sugar-filled culprits like candy, soft drinks, cereals, cookies, and cakes. However, if you read all the labels on your packaged foods, you may be surprised to find just how sneaky manufacturers are. Sugar is in soups, breads, condiments, health foods, salad dressings, and even rotisserie chicken!

Finding sugar can be tricky, too, because it has multiple names. Look for:

- Sugar

- Honey

- Agave

- Corn sweetener, corn syrup

- Fruit juice concentrates

- Invert sugar

- Malt sugar

- Molasses

- Sugar code names ending in "ose" (dextrose, fructose, glucose, lactose, maltose, sucralose)

MORE TIPS AND TRICKS
TO LOSE WEIGHT

Outside of intermittent fasting, ensuring you are properly hydrated, and avoiding added sugars, here's what else we know works for everyone to lose weight:

- Eat foods as close to their natural state as possible. That means keep processed foods to a minimum. Think about it like this, if you're buying items that are *not* on the perimeter of the grocery store, it is processed in some way. Steer clear of those inner aisles as much as possible!

- Don't over-stress your body with workouts! Remember, over-exercising can be a stressor. Your workouts should invigorate you, not exhaust you or stress your body too much. Over-training or obsessing about working out also causes an imbalance in the body, adding to stress and cortisol levels. Remember, balance is the key. Listen and tune in to your body and how you are feeling. If you ever think you're over-doing it in the gym or on the track, you probably are.

- Get enough sleep! This is a big one for most of us. We are often up late watching TV or on the computer, the light of which stimulates the brain and makes it difficult to fall asleep once we're in bed. And your daily Frappuccino pick-me-up in the afternoon can be a problem for your sleep in the evening! Caffeine consumed during the day is still in our bloodstream up to twelve hours later. And research shows that proper sleep leads to less snacking on junk food, more weight loss during dieting, and regulated and efficient metabolism.[41]

- Don't allow yourself two "cheats" in a row. Brandon Zenisek, in our office, calls this "stacking." Stacking two "cheats" in a row can start momentum for another. However, do stack as many healthier meals as you want to build momentum that way. So, if you have a less-than-healthy breakfast (like a big burrito loaded with several eggs, cheese, and sausage, or a stack of pancakes), then try to have a clean lunch. Or, if you have ice cream or some other decadent desert after a big dinner, then consider fasting for breakfast the next day or keeping it on the lighter side with a few eggs or Greek yogurt with some berries. It's very easy to keep sliding once you allow a cheat!

- On a related note, we suggest you "treat treats as treats." Remember, treats should be something special you indulge in on the rare or special occasion. Because there is such an abundance of premade bakery items available, it's easy to think it's normal to have them every day. But try to remember to stop and think before you have one. They are meant for special occasions. Just because they are in sealed single-serving packages doesn't mean it's a special occasion!

There should be a place for cheesecake or a sweet in your healthy nutritional habits, but having a piece of cheesecake every night is no longer treating a treat like a treat.

- Weigh yourself every day using a scale that gives you more information than just your weight. These scales can be inexpensive (on Amazon, they have them for around fifteen dollars). But the information they provide you is priceless. Additionally, as mentioned in Chapter 5, there are some great biometric body composition scales available with electric impedance technology that will provide the best and most insightful data you can use regarding your health and weight. We suggest you always weigh yourself first thing in the morning, right after you use the restroom. Do not eat or drink anything before stepping on the scale, and wear the same clothing (or nothing) each time.

- Take time every day to celebrate non-scale victories. Did you choose fresh berries instead of ice cream for dessert? Celebrate yourself! Did you sit on the floor and get back up without getting a boost? Celebrate it!

- Store processed food and junk foods in a closet or out-of-the way place that's hard to reach. One of our clients actually put those foods in the laundry room to make it inconvenient for everyone in her family. Sometimes out-of-sight-out-of-mind works!

- Conversely, in-sight-in-mind also works. When you come home from the market, before you put your vegetables away, prep them to be easy-access snacks. Clean and cut them into small pieces, maybe sprinkle a little seasoning on them, then store them in the refrigerator at eye-level in clear containers.

- Similarly, pre-wash most of your fruits so they are at the ready. We say "most" and not all, because pre-washing berries will make them rot faster.

- Make a large batch of salad—cut up lettuces, tomatoes, cucumber, onion, carrots, and celery—and keep it stored in the refrigerator so you always have a quick salad on hand.

- To encourage yourself to eat less, use a medium-sized plate. It may sound silly, but there is research that shows we eat less when we use smaller plates or dishes.[42]

- When you are going to a big event or a party, fill yourself up before you go with a large salad or some lean protein. This will prevent you from being hungry when they are serving all those finger foods and hor d'oeurves, which are very easy to overindulge on!

- Remember: hydration is important! Make the first liquid you drink each morning be plain water—yes, before your coffee and tea.

- If you are a fan of breakfast, choose foods that are *not* based on refined carbohydrates—eliminate most cereals, breads, and pastries. Most of us are pretty sedentary after breakfast. We sit in our cars as we drive to work, then sit behind a desk. That means those fast-acting carbohydrates get converted to sugar for fuel you don't really need, so you wind up storing it as fat on your body. Then, with no energy left, you are super hungry at lunch. Because it takes longer for lean protein to be broken down and used for energy, it supplies a slow release of fuel over the course of your day and makes you less hungry at lunch.

- Get some kind of movement every day! We're not talking going to the gym and lifting weights for ninety minutes. Just walk every day, preferably for an hour, which you can break up if you need to. Get fifteen minutes in before work, another fifteen after work, then a half hour after dinner. If the weather is bad outside, you can spend your half-hour marching in place as you watch TV if you need to.

- Keep a food journal that records how you feel, what you weigh, and how you slept after you eat a certain kind of food. Sometimes, the effects may not be noticed until the next day, and often these records will surprise you. Note any stomach distress, episodes of fatigue, headaches, joint or muscle pain, and weight fluctuations. Then make a habit of reviewing your journal on a weekly basis to look for trends.

You might be surprised by what you find! Dan thought the first time he gained two pounds the day after eating Greek yogurt was a fluke. But after noticing it happening several times, he realized there's something about that food that kicks in his inflammatory response. So he avoids it now.

- When ordering at a restaurant, always get the dressing on the side. But here's something even better to remember when at a restaurant: if you tell them you have "dietary restrictions," (for example, if you're trying to remove fats or oils), they will be happier to go out of their way to make a good meal with other options than if you just say, "I'm on a diet."

- Tap into the power of positivity each day. Spend a few minutes before bed writing in a gratitude journal, or take sixty seconds to sit in quiet reflection before you begin eating your meals. However you do it, find time every day to appreciate your efforts to take good care of your body, tune in to how good your body feels when you eat healthy foods. You can even take it further and think about how many people and events had to transpire to get the seeds of the food planted, then nurtured to grow, then harvested, packaged, transported to a distributor, transported to a grocer, placed on shelves, etc.—all for you to enjoy and nourish your body. It's pretty amazing when you think about it. Express your gratitude for it!

Now that you're armed with some handy behaviors that can help you lose weight and keep it off, let's discuss the kinds of foods most people do well with on their weight loss journey.

CHAPTER 7

EATING
LIKE A PRO

Stuart had always been on the bigger side, but it never really interfered with his life. However, as he grew older, his size increased, and it started slowing him down. As with many people who gain weight as they age, he developed type 2 diabetes and then arthritis in his back. With help from his general practitioner, he managed to get the diabetes controlled through medication, but the arthritis is in an area of his spine that makes his legs hurt when he exerts them in any way. Just doing some light gardening caused him agony.

The pain in his legs was his primary reason for wanting to lose weight, but our nutritional approach is what prompted him come to *re:vitalize* for help losing it. Stuart had tried numerous other plans in the past, including a brand-name program that required him to eat their powdered shakes and bars. He lasted for two years on that plan, eating two meals a day based on their shakes and bars, and then one meal of lean proteins and green vegetables.

He lost a little weight, but he was perfectly miserable the entire time. Not only was the food limited, it was not satisfying. He grew bored with it in just a couple of weeks, and, worse, he was hungry non-stop. The plan was just too extreme for him—we think it's too limiting and extreme for anyone who needs to be on a plan for longer than a week or two. And unfortunately, the plan backfired. His weight ballooned soon after he went off the plan and began eating regular food again.

Client Body Composition Biodata: Before and After Results

Stuart	57 yo	6' 6"	Male			
	Before	After	Difference
Weight	392.6	333.4	-59.2
BMI Change/Improvement			-6.9
Body Fat % Lost			-2.3%
Visceral Fat Rating Improvement			-5

Stuart wanted a plan where he could lose weight while not feeling hungry. And that's what he got when he came to *re:vitalize*. After his initial consult appointment with us, we gave him a list of the foods he would be eating for the next forty days and provided some recipes and menu suggestions so that he'd be satisfied and fulfilled. We encouraged him, as we do all our clients, to let us know if he ever felt hungry or weak so we can help him. Those are signs of not giving your body what it needs, which is *not* a healthy way to lose weight or do anything else.

Stuart said, "You had me at 'real food,'" and signed on with the program. Soon, he was coming in for his weekly check-ins. At each visit he reported how he felt better overall. He started sleeping better. His energy improved. Even his libido picked up. As the weight came off, his legs hurt less. And he wasn't hungry, nor was he bored with the foods.

EAT "REAL" FOOD
AND STILL LOSE WEIGHT.

I f losing weight was merely about calories-in-calories-out, figuring out the best foods for everyone would be a simple matter. Dan and I would give you a list of foods and their calories and provide a list of exercises to go with it, with the math calculating how to burn the excess calories.

However, we know it's not that simple. Stress, you know by now, is one big reason why it's not that easy. And our age really does play a role, as Stuart experienced. The thing is, as we age, it becomes even more important that we get the right nutrition for our bodies, which is another reason why we find "real" food to be preferable.

See, one of the things that happen as we grow older is we begin losing digestive enzymes, which are secretions our body produces to help us get the nutrients out of our foods.[43] Your pancreas is the main digestive enzyme factory in your body, but your salivary glands, stomach, and intestines also produce them. When you eat something, different enzymes are used to break the food down into molecules so your body can get the nutrition it needs. Here are the main ones:

- Lipase: breaks down fats.

- Protease: breaks down proteins.

- Amylase: breaks down carbohydrates.

In addition to those are numerous other ones like lactase, which breaks down lactose, the sugar in milk. So you can see, if you don't have the digestive enzymes you need, you will not be able to process your foods to get the nutrient goodies they provide. Instead, what happens to many people is they suffer upset stomachs, gas and bloating, irritable bowels, and other intestinal distress.

So, if we lose our enzymes as we age, that means we will not be able to assimilate or metabolize foods as well we did when we were young. To counter that, many people take digestive enzyme supplements with their food (please, discuss any kind of supplementation with your doctor). However, if you read on the bottles of those supplements, you'll discover that many of them are made with plants! Papayas, bananas, avocados, mangoes, and fermented foods like kimchi are loaded with digestive enzymes, *and* they are healthy for you!

"It's important at any age to have vitamins and minerals, but much more important as we age so these enzymes work together with these vital nutrients. Supplementing digestive enzymes becomes important because, as we age, we have a decreased ability to digest, absorb, and metabolize nutrients. Depending on the type of medications you're taking (or have taken), these deplete nutrients in the body, which is why supplementation is so necessary. This is why digestive problems are so common among people over 60. Half the people over 60 don't make enough stomach acid to digest their food adequately. Supplementing digestive enzymes can help your body process food efficiently."

—DR. PATRICK PORTER, PH.D.[44]

In other words, digestive enzymes are just *one* more reason why we always think real food is best for everyone. Protein powders, shakes, and bars just don't have everything your body needs for optimum health—which is always part of the goal for our patients: lose weight *and* be healthy.

But, while real food is best, not everyone can eat the same stuff and get the same results. That's why we always do a complete bioscan and create a nutritional profile for each of our clients. However, there are some foods that seem to work for most people. So consider the following as generalized, loose guidance about what we think *most* people can eat and find an improvement in their weight and overall health.

MEET PHYTONUTRIENTS

We like taking a paleo-vegan approach to eating. Dr. Mark Hyman calls it "Pegan." We like it because it seems to provide the foods that most nutritional research suggests we need. In short, a paleo-vegan diet is:

- High in vegetables and fruits

- Low-glycemic, meaning there is little to no sugar, refined flour, or other refined carbohydrates like pasta, rice, bread, etc., the majority of the time.

- Enough protein but not too much. We should all aim for .4 grams of protein per pound of body weight each day. To give you an idea of what that looks like on your plate, that translates into 60 grams for someone who weighs 150 pounds. For perspective, a chicken breast with the bone and skin removed, on average, has about 27 grams of protein, and four ounces of steak has about 28 grams. One serving (about 4 ounces) of an animal protein source will give you half of what your body needs for protein each day. This may seem like a shockingly low amount of protein meat, but in reality, our plates should be largely plants, and meat should be the garnish.

- An emphasis on chemical-free foods (no preservatives or artificial sweeteners) that are ideally organic.

Choosing foods to eat along that nutritional guidance will provide not only adequate nutrition from your basic vitamins and minerals, but you will also gain the benefit of getting the micronutrients and phytonutrients from your foods. These nutrients are impossible to get in refined or processed items because the act of refining and processing strips those nutrients out of the food.

Micronutrients and phytonutrients are a big deal! They are also called phytochemicals because they don't technically supply energy, but they do supply an amazing amount of health benefits to us. Phytonutrients are found in plant, where they act as defenders to help those plants survive disease or even insect infestations. When we eat those plants and consume the phytonutrients as well, we benefit.

Phytonutrients are powerful antioxidants, which helps us fight illnesses and disease. They have been known to help decrease blood pressure and cholesterol, to reduce symptoms from menopause, and to lessen the risk of osteoporosis. They're beneficial to our eyesight in that they prevent cataracts, and some have been found to reduce the probability of certain cancers forming.[45]

And here's something that sounds kind of crazy: just one piece of fruit or vegetable may contain more than fifty phytochemicals!

When you eat your fruits and vegetables, you get the best nutrition. You also can eat more, get full, and not have to worry about your weight. Think about it: one candy bar typically has about 120 calories in it. To get 120 calories from vegetables, you would have to eat one of the following:

- 4 cups of kale

- 12 stalks of celery

- 4 carrots

- 30 spears of asparagus!

- 2½ stalks of broccoli

- 12 cucumbers

- 4½ cups of snap beans

- 2 heads of iceberg lettuce

- 4½ medium-sized tomatoes

Who can eat 12 stalks of celery at one time? Not many—if any—humans! One or two will make you feel full and satisfied, and with all the fiber you get from them, you'll be satisfied much longer than you will after that sugar spike from your candy bar drops.

But we don't just recommend eating fruits and vegetables for weight loss. Remember the beginning of the book when we learned how our livers can have trouble detoxing? Well, there are actually foods that help your liver do its detoxification job.

FOODS THAT
SUPPORT DETOXIFICATION

There are numerous detox diets on the market that claim to eliminate toxins and improve your health, as well as promote weight loss. Usually, these diets rely on an herbal mixture while you fast for a couple of days. One of them encourages you to eat or drink nothing but hot water, lemon, and honey!

While each has raving fans and proponents who swear by their effectiveness, we like to take a gentler, easier approach to detoxification. And since our bodies are already designed to have all the necessary equipment to detox (kidneys, liver, and the lymphatic system), all we need to do is let them do their jobs. We can, though, make things easier on our bodies by *not* loading up with an imbalance of processed foods. Additionally, if our staff at our clinics suspect a client is storing toxins, we may encourage them to eat particular foods as well as take supplements that support our bodies' detoxification mechanisms. And you know what? You may already be eating some of these on a regular basis, anyway. Just choosing to eat more of them and less of non-organic foods and processed foods will do your liver a huge favor.

Here are some of our favorite foods that are also natural detoxers.

Apples

This common fruit is loaded with pectin, a fiber that helps remove toxins and cholesterol from your blood, and malic acid, which is reported to soften gallstones and help your body rid itself of heavy metals.

Artichokes

They may be hard to figure out how to eat, but it's worth the effort! Artichokes are loaded with fiber and antioxidants that stimulate the liver's detox methods and help us digest fatty foods to eliminate the toxins.

Cabbage

Not just cabbage, but most of the cruciferous vegetables (broccoli, cauliflower, and kale) contain a chemical called sulforaphane, which is a detoxing agent. Cabbage also has glutathione, which is an antioxidant that actually helps the body bind toxins to make them available for elimination.

Citrus Fruits

We're particularly talking about lemons, here, but to some extent limes and oranges, too. These fruits are loaded with vitamin C, which is an antioxidant that fights free-radicals (which are cancer- and disease-causing compounds) in your body. As far as detoxing goes, though, the citric acid in lemons contain d-limonene, a chemical that helps the liver break down toxic substances.

Chlorella and Spirulina

You'd be forgiven if these words sound more like space alien names! Not many people have heard of them. And if they have, would know they are forms of algae and wonder what's so great about them! Well, here's what's so great: they are both considered superfoods because they pack a powerful amount of nutrients in a tiny amount of food. Yes, they're loaded with phytonutrients, but also have amino acids, magnesium, a host of B vitamins, potassium, and more. And as far as detoxing goes, they are natural chelators, which means they remove heavy metals from our bodies. And spirulina is good for eliminating arsenic.

Arsenic has nothing to do with old lace!

In 2016, the FDA released a report on arsenic in rice and rice products. While it set off a legitimate maelstrom of concern about the safety of everyday foods (including baby foods), most of us aren't aware of just how much we're exposed to arsenic.

It's a naturally occurring element in our soils, water, and even air (volcanic eruptions can force massive quantities into the air). When it's naturally occurring in the soil or being spewed into the air, it's a less toxic form of arsenic than the inorganic forms of arsenic that come from fracking, coal-fired plants, mining, arsenic-treated lumber, and pesticides.

For some reason, seafood is more prone to absorbing the naturally occurring arsenic, and rice is highly susceptible to accumulating the inorganic, toxic arsenic.

So, if you eat rice or rice products (rice milk, cereals, and nutritional bars) on a regular basis, consider experimenting with spirulina as a seasoning.

Greens

Probably the most passed section of the produce department in supermarkets is the one containing greens. Other than parsley, not many people approach or even know what to do with bitters, dandelion, arugula, and many of the other dark, green leafy vegetables. However, be brave and dabble in them! They have high levels of chlorophyl, which is a super detoxification agent.

Spices

Turmeric and ginger are known anti-inflammatories, which we all could use more of. But they also contain curcumin in turmeric, which supports the gallbladder by encouraging it to produce more bile. In turn, bile helps cleanse your liver and prevents toxins from damaging it. Meanwhile, ginger assists your elimination pathways by stimulating digestion and sweating.

Watercress

It might be surprising to learn that watercress is one of the healthiest foods to eat! They include lots of B vitamins, which are needed for the process that transforms toxins into being water soluble in order for us to eliminate them. Watercress also has antioxidants, zinc, potassium, and other minerals. In addition, it's a diuretic, which means after making the toxins water soluble, we can easily and quickly eliminate them.

While all the above foods help with detoxing, which will help with weight loss, we also need to talk about what to do with all the inflammation in our bodies. We've already mentioned that belly fat sends out chemicals that encourages painful inflammation, which is not necessarily good news. However, what is good news is that healthy eating can be anti-inflammatory, which will encourage easier digestion and more physical movement—both things necessary for weight loss.

ANTI-INFLAMMATORY
FOODS

Here are our top ten anti-inflammatory foods:

1. Berries. All of them! Strawberries, raspberries, blackberries, boysenberries, and blueberries.

2. Fatty fish like salmon, sardines, herring, mackerel, and anchovies. They all have omega-3 fatty acids in them that are powerful antioxidants. But fish can be loaded with heavy metals, so try not to overload on them. Find wild-caught species as they tend to have less mercury than farm-raised fish.

3. Avocados and Extra Virgin Olive Oil. Two more sources of healthy fats, both of which inhibit inflammation. One of our favorite tricks is to replace butter on toast with avocados. Yum!

4. Green tea. There is something called epigallocatechin-3-gallate (EGCG) in green tea that reduces pro-inflammatory cytokine production.

5. Peppers. All varieties of bell peppers and chili peppers are loaded with vitamin C and antioxidants that produce anti-inflammatory effects. However, bell peppers go one step further. They pack a punch with quercetin, which can reduce damage in people with sarcoidosis, an inflammatory disease.

6. Mushrooms. With studies showing cooking reduces their phenols and other antioxidants that give them anti-inflammatory properties, we recommend eating your mushrooms raw or just lightly cooked.

7. Grapes. This fruit contains anthocyanins, which reduce inflammation.

8. Dark chocolate and cocoa. Finally! Something sounding like dessert is healthy! Yes, dark chocolate has antioxidants that reduce inflammation and are suspected of reducing your risk of getting any disease, thus leading to healthier aging. It's the flavanols in chocolate that are responsible for all the good they do.

9. Tomatoes. High in vitamin C and potassium, these fruits (right, they're *not* vegetables) also contain lycopene, an antioxidant with anti-inflammatory properties.

10. Cherries. This tiny fruit has a huge benefit: it's rich in antioxidants, like anthocyanins and catechins, that fight inflammation.

Hopefully, the lists of detoxing foods and anti-inflammatory foods show you that you can eat good-tasting foods that do good for your body as you try to lose and maintain your weight. But what if you find yourself with strong cravings for something you know you shouldn't have—at least not while you're trying to lose? What do you do then?

MANAGING CRAVINGS

A s with many in the weight loss community, we used to rely solely on what's commonly called the Four Ds to overcome cravings. They are:

1. **Delay.** Tell yourself after twenty minutes, or after the next commercial break, or after whatever, that if you are still craving the food, you'll indulge—just a little. Then, drink a full glass of water and set a timer if you need to. We don't think the timer is a good thing because often if you can distract yourself enough during those twenty minutes, you'll forget about the craving. If so, the timer may accidentally make you remember and start it all over again.

2. **Determine.** Get to the root reason of why you want the food you're craving. Is there something else you need that could satiate that craving—emotionally, physically, or nutritionally? Often, when we need a nap, we'll crave carbohydrates. Or when we want "something crunchy," we're really just bored. As we spoke about early in the book, sometimes stress sets out that ghrelin signal telling us to eat something sweet to give us fuel, when we really don't need it. Perhaps a mindfulness exercise or some other form of stress release would do the trick.

3. **Distract.** Some call this tactic "urge-surfing," which we like to use. In essence, it just means do something else to distract you from the craving. Just take ten minutes to go for a short walk, do some push-ups, clean out the junk drawer, anything that requires you to pay attention to something else.

4. **Distance.** Remember that tip about putting the junk food where it's hard to reach? Well, if it still feels too close when you have a craving, leave the room! Leave the building if you have to. Get yourself as far away from it as possible until the craving passes.

While the above tactics are helpful, we can't forget something important about your cravings. They could be telling you that you are missing an important nutrient. If that's the case, check out the graphic below to see what healthy, low-calorie option you have to fulfill that need.

How To Beat Food Cravings

revitalizeweightloss.com

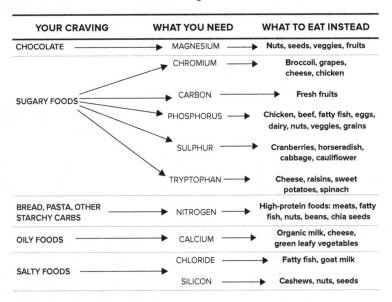

YOUR CRAVING	WHAT YOU NEED	WHAT TO EAT INSTEAD
CHOCOLATE	MAGNESIUM	Nuts, seeds, veggies, fruits
SUGARY FOODS	CHROMIUM	Broccoli, grapes, cheese, chicken
	CARBON	Fresh fruits
	PHOSPHORUS	Chicken, beef, fatty fish, eggs, dairy, nuts, veggies, grains
	SULPHUR	Cranberries, horseradish, cabbage, cauliflower
	TRYPTOPHAN	Cheese, raisins, sweet potatoes, spinach
BREAD, PASTA, OTHER STARCHY CARBS	NITROGEN	High-protein foods: meats, fatty fish, nuts, beans, chia seeds
OILY FOODS	CALCIUM	Organic milk, cheese, green leafy vegetables
SALTY FOODS	CHLORIDE	Fatty fish, goat milk
	SILICON	Cashews, nuts, seeds

Source: Coaching & Weight Management

Of course, there are times when it's OK to give into your cravings.
But be mindful when you do. Make sure you enjoy them and don't
overindulge so much that you regret it the next morning when you
get on the scale.

Now you have some techniques to lose weight and some good foods
to help you do so. But if you want more help and more structure,
turn the page to see how we use this information to tackle weight
loss for our clients.

CHAPTER 8

HOW WE DO IT

Larry's shoulder hurt, but he didn't pay too much attention. He was a busy guy—working twelve-hour days Monday through Thursday, then going over to his mother's house to give his sister a break from caregiving. He'd spend Thursday night through Monday morning taking care of his mother, who was bedridden with illness.

He held that routine for almost two years, coping with it by eating on the road, usually from fast-food places, and drinking copious amounts of his favorite drink: Frappuccinos. When his mother passed away, he was hooked on caffeine and dangerously overweight, at 438 pounds.

At that point, he finally went to the doctor to check out his shoulder. He needed to have rotator cuff surgery. As the former team physician for the Milwaukee Brewers and Phoenix Suns, Dr. Tom Fiel easily recognized the problem with Larry's shoulder. But Dr. Fiel thought Larry had a bigger concern: his weight. Larry agreed he had a problem with it. He was much bigger than he wanted to be, and he wasn't getting much joy out of life because of it.

So he quit drinking soda and switched from his beloved Frappuccinos to water and coffee—though it was still loaded vanilla creamer. Some serious weight came off; he dropped down to 315 pounds. However, at a follow-up visit, his doctor scared him: he had type 2 diabetes.

Larry was never a fan of pharmaceuticals, so he resisted the doctor's attempts to put him on medication to control his diabetes. But he had trouble losing the weight, and the diabetes started winning. He developed neuropathy in his feet and started noticing other changes in his body.

He tried going to a nutritionist, who greeted him with, "You're severely obese." He felt shamed, not encouraged, and tuned her out. His next stop was to our clinic where he was greeted for what he is: a valuable human being whose body needed to find balance.

Dan took his biometrics and explained to him the science behind what we do. He felt educated, and the nutritional plan made sense to him, so he gladly began. Six months later he shocked his doctor at his follow-up visit. Not only his weight had come down, but his blood sugar was beginning to stabilize, too.

Client Body Composition Biodata: Before and After Results

Larry	56 yo | 6' 0" | Male		
	Before	**After**	**Difference**
Weight	297.2	258	-39.2
BMI Change/Improvement			-5.3
Body Fat % Lost			-9.1%
Visceral Fat Rating Improvement			-6.4
Cellular Hydration Improvement[1]			+6.3%
Metabolic Improvement[2]			-31 yrs

[1] Change in body water %
[2] As measured by metabolic age reversal/improvement

OUR METHODOLOGY TO FIND BALANCE

The re:vitalize 4 Stage Weight Loss Roadmap

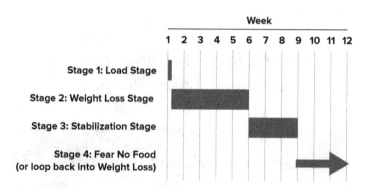

Larry was impressed by the way we explained the science behind weight loss and the tools we use to help people in our clinics. We've heard it said more than once that "losing weight isn't rocket science," and we agree each time—rocket science is much easier! Rocket science requires math that is the same no matter who uses it. There is less variation and unpredictability in how rockets are made than in the way the human body functions (or malfunctions).

But we do have tools to make it easier to figure out how to make weight loss happen. One of those tools allows us to do a full biometric scan to get a body composition and metabolic analysis of *you*. That biodata will give us your body fat percentage, hydration levels, muscle mass amount, visceral fat amount, and metabolic age (among other points of biodata).

Next comes the bioscan technology that will generate your customized micronutrient profile. That tells us the vitamins, minerals, and phytonutrients that your body may benefit from to bring it back into balance to help fix your metabolism. It also allows our clients to make better food choices because it will tell us which foods are optimal for weight loss for each individual. As you know, no two bodies are identical. So, while there are some foods that your sister, brother, parent, aunt, uncle, or best friend can eat and never gain an ounce from, those foods may do the opposite for you—and vice versa. And our bioscan technology can help you figure out which foods will assimilate better with *your* metabolism. Then, armed with that knowledge, we compile a list of foods and supplements that will give *you* the specific nutrients *you* need.

> Doc and Dan Do: eat what's right for you! We used our bioscan technology to help us see which foods could be optimized for our weight loss and which foods work best with our metabolism.

At that point, you'll have a plan. Typically, we create a plan for you that extends over four stages. Each one is specifically designed to deconstruct and change habits, address micronutrient deficiencies and imbalances affecting metabolic function, and of course lose body fat. Our team will outline for you the general pillars for each stage and how they will work so you can try them at home. The specifics and duration of these stages will be guided by your unique bioscan food and supplement protocols and our expert nutrition team, so, while you can go through the stages without us, if you want a customized roadmap, you should schedule a consultation.

Stage One

You start out in our "load stage," which only lasts for one day. On this day, you'll eat whatever you want as long as you get in two or three healthy fats. As you'll see in the next stage, you will eliminate all fats and oils for a period of time, so we want you to load up on them now:

- Avocado or guacamole

- Fatty fish like salmon or Ahi tuna—get that sushi in!

- Olive oil

- Raw nuts

- Grass-fed beef and the butter that comes from them.

We remind people that since they may not be able to eat their favorite foods for a little while (pizza, ice cream, nachos, etc.), and they should eat it as a celebration to start their plan.

Beginning in stage one, we will also start you on your specific supplement protocol to get your body acclimated to taking the supplements. For any readers who haven't gone through a bioscan from *re:vitalize*, we generally recommend a high-quality electrolyte trace mineral supplement as well as a molecular hydrogen supplement—like our Mineral:Pure and Hydro:Active products—to aid in hydration and metabolic repair (as we spoke about in Chapter 6).

Stage Two

Next is the lose-it stage. The length of it will vary depending on what your profile suggests you need and the amount of weight you want to lose. Typically, it lasts between twenty and forty days. Frankly, we do *not* recommend that people stay on it for more than forty days because you do eliminate, as much as possible, fats and oils from your diet. And you need them. So you can't go for too long without them.

This stage is when your body will heal. It will be in a constant anti-inflammatory and detoxifying state, while you fuel yourself with a wide spectrum of healthy, whole foods and micronutrients that aid in everything you want it to: metabolic repair, hormonal balancing, and weight loss. So, yes, this is an exciting stage!

You will lose a large amount of fat and begin to see and feel the difference in your body as you detox, heal, and rebalance. But be forewarned: stage two is simple, but simple doesn't always mean easy.

You might bump into a few cravings or find you're more entrenched in old habits than you thought you were. We promise, though, that the cravings *will* go away as your body rebalances and new habits set into place. And the best part: now is when you create the foundation for new healthy habits. Your awareness of what you eat and how you feel in response to it increases, as does your taste preference for veggies and the natural sugars in fruit. It is during this stage that your body adjusts to and learns to feel truly satiated on unprocessed foods.

Having an accountability buddy or support from someone who understands what you're going through is very important during this stage. Many of our clients have told us that because they know everyone on our staff has done the program—so they *truly* understand and can genuinely empathize—really helps them. (And we've found some delicious work arounds for staying on track and really enjoying food while on the program.)

During this time, you will need to weigh yourself every day on a digital scale that measures to the tenths of a pound so you can be sure you are losing. That's the easy part.

You will also need to choose your eating window, because intermittent fasting is necessary for this phase. During this window, you will eat two meals of vegetables and protein and have two snacks of fruit. If you get hungry in between, you can snack on more vegetables because guess what? There's no calorie counting! And because one of the benefits of the biometrics we take on you is that we can identify the foods that will satisfy you so that you're not hungry during this stage!

You will need to eliminate all sorts of fats from your diet. This even includes those healthy oils and healthy high-fat foods we love, like olive and coconut oils, nuts, seeds, avocados, etc. *But wait!* We can hear you challenging us already. You're wondering: *aren't healthy fats and oils good for you?*

Yep, they sure are, which is why we bring those back into the diet with a vengeance a little later. It's just that during the initial weight loss stage of our program, by limiting the fat in your diet, we're better able to jump-start the reboot of your metabolism and get your body to use your fat stores for fuel.

Many consider this to be the most challenging part of the program because we rely heavily on fats and oils to cook. But there are a few alternatives you can try. One is to experiment with coconut aminos or liquid aminos to keep foods from sticking to pans. Mushroom broth or organic chicken broth works well. These products will give a nice flavor to your foods, too. Also, consider investing in an air fryer. They're a great option as they allow you to cook almost anything oil free.

If you will be eating out, you'll need to remember to ask the restaurant to prepare your meal without oils or butters, and tell them it's because of a "dietary restriction." And just as with sugar, read the ingredient lists on labels. Many processed, preprepared foods will contain added fat or oil. Our intention is not to make you fear fats and oils—remember, our motto is Fear No Food. Healthy fats and oils are integral for a fully nutritional way of eating. Fats fuel our bodies and our brains, but you can safely take some time off from them during this stage—and you should, if you want to be successful on this program.

Although you'll be eliminating fat in this stage, you'll be adding in vegetables—lots and lots of vegetables. In fact, we ask that you eat at least a pound of vegetables every day—the ones that your bioscan suggests you need. But again, we promise you, you won't be hungry! And you'll be fulfilling some holes in your nutritional makeup, so you won't be craving anything either.

You will not be able to eat any sugar during this stage, which probably doesn't surprise you. But you can use stevia to sweeten your (black) coffee or tea, and you will drink a lot of water. We'll also suggest some supplementation that will help your water actually hydrate you. Stage two is not always easy, but your body will feel so much better!

Foods for Stage Two

While the following list isn't personalized to you, these are foods that we find most people can eat during this stage:

Proteins (serving sizes: three-to-four-ounce servings for land animals; five to six ounces for seafood. Eggs are two whole egg or one whole egg with three egg whites):

✓ Eggs	✓ Lobster
✓ Cod	✓ Scallop
✓ Flounder	✓ Shrimp
✓ Haddock	✓ Chicken
✓ Halibut	✓ Turkey
✓ Mahi Mahi	✓ Lean Beef
✓ Tilapia	✓ Buffalo
✓ Crab	

Vegetables (no maximum! Eat sixteen to twenty ounces a day):

✓ Alfalfa	✓ Kale
✓ Asparagus	✓ Leek
✓ Artichoke	✓ Lettuce

- ✓ Broccoli (no more than once per week)
- ✓ Brussels sprouts
- ✓ Cabbage
- ✓ Cauliflower (no more than once per week)
- ✓ Celery
- ✓ Chard
- ✓ Collard greens
- ✓ Cucumber
- ✓ Fennel
- ✓ Mushroom
- ✓ Onion
- ✓ Peppers
- ✓ Radish
- ✓ Shallots
- ✓ Spinach
- ✓ String Beans
- ✓ Zucchini

Fruits:

- ✓ Apple
- ✓ Apricot
- ✓ Blackberry (½ cup)
- ✓ Blueberry (½ cup)
- ✓ Cherry (½ cup)
- ✓ Grapefruit (½)
- ✓ Lemon
- ✓ Lime
- ✓ Orange
- ✓ Peach (½)
- ✓ Pear
- ✓ Plum
- ✓ Raspberry (½ cup)
- ✓ Strawberry (1 cup, halved)
- ✓ Watermelon (1 cup, cubed)

Vegetarian and Vegan Options

Meat Substitutes:

- ✓ Beyond Meat Burgers (1 patty)

- ✓ Hillary's Veggie Burger (1 patty)

- ✓ Tofu (6 ounces)

Protein Powder:

- ✓ Garden of Life Vegan Protein Powder (Sport or Protein & Greens)

- ✓ Hemp Yeah! (Unsweetened only)

- ✓ Vega (Sport Premium, Clean Protein, or Protein & Greens)

Dairy-Based Protein:

- ✓ Eggs (2 whole OR 3 egg whites plus 1 whole egg)

- ✓ Low-fat plain kefir (1 cup)

- ✓ Low-fat cottage cheese (1 cup)

- ✓ Plain low-fat or Greek yogurt (1 cup)

Vegan:

- ✓ Dairy-free yogurt (1 cup)—LAWA, Cocoyo, Forager brands, and Kite Hill are good (unsweetened or unsweetened vanilla)

✓ Chia seeds (2 tbs)

✓ Black beans (½ cup)

✓ Lentils (½ cup)

✓ Spirulina (2 tbs)

✓ Quinoa (1 cup)

✓ Chickpeas (½ cup)

Plateaus

To ensure that your weight loss remains consistent and that you continue to build the momentum of seeing the numbers go down on your scale just about every day, we have several tactics to help move you off a plateau quickly. With traditional dieting, plateaus can last anywhere from two to six weeks or more, which can be very frustrating, especially when you're doing all the right things.

So, if your weight loss has stagnated for more than three days, here are a few reset strategies to restart that metabolism burn:

Protein Day:

Spend one day fasting until dinner (usually around four or five o'clock in the evening) then eat six ounces of a land protein OR eight ounces of a sea protein. Sorry, no eggs or cottage cheese for this meal! Pair your protein with either a raw tomato or an organic apple. Be sure to drink plenty of water with electrolytes in it and take a mineral supplement. The lean protein will up-regulate an important pathway of cellular energy regulation called the AMP-activated protein kinase pathway. This, in turn, promotes lipid metabolism, which means your body will release stored fats to provide you with energy. Protein day also supports stable blood sugar and insulin release.

Apple Day:

Eat only apples for one day. A day of apples works in two different ways to reset your weight. First, apples are loaded with pectin, which is a starch that may prevent degradation to the liver so it can perform its many functions well. And the liver is a workhorse! One of the things it does is filter the blood to detox the body. Consuming only apples for a day positively impacts the liver by supplying a plentitude of pectin. The second way a day of apples resets you is that they primarily consist of simple carbohydrates, which are easily digested and absorbed by the body to utilize as energy. Because the liver plays a large role in the metabolism of more complex macronutrients, this consumption of isolated simple sugars puts minimal pressure on the liver metabolically, making it more effective.

Raw Vegetable Day:

Similar to apple day, spending a day eating only RAW vegetables will take a great amount of pressure off of your liver so it can more easily carry out basic metabolic pathways. Additionally, various kinds of vegetables (cruciferous in particular) have been found in studies to modulate the activity of liver enzymes directly involved in detoxification processes.[46] This implies that raw vegetable day could enable the liver to become more efficient at detoxing.

Eggs, Coconut Oil, and Coffee Day:

Like the meat consumed on a protein day, eggs are a high-quality form of protein that can promote fat breakdown by stimulating an energy regulation pathway in cells. By cooking your eggs in coconut oil, you will also influence lipid metabolism. Coconut oil is classified as a medium-chained triglyceride (MCT), a type of fat structure that is more readily digested, absorbed, and utilized as an energy source than other types of fat. Therefore, they are less likely to be stored as fat. Additionally, specific fatty acids (oleic acid in particular) that coconut oil contains can potentially induce lipolysis and regulate lipid metabolism.

You can eat up to four eggs fried in one tablespoon of coconut oil in the morning. Then, enjoy two cups of coffee blended with one tablespoon each of coconut oil throughout the day. Try it with our English toffee stevia—it's amazing!

In case you're wondering how reset days work, they do so by contributing to systems, processes, and internal environments that precede initiation of lipolysis and beta-oxidation. In other words, although a caloric deficit exists for each reset day, and that alone can be a reason behind the large drops in weight, there is more going on at a cellular level that kind of tricks your body into revving your metabolism.

Stage Three

As you move into stage three, you move from a high-structure-with-high-support stage to a high-structure-with-less-support one, and you will open the guard rails and begin to reintroduce other food groups. By now, you will have learned a little about nutrition and started forging healthier habits, like incorporating vegetables into your diet every day. And, most excitedly, you are seeing the effects of those healthier habits on your body and mindset. Not only have you lost weight and found improved energy levels, but you've probably noticed better moods and sleep, and an even enhanced libido.

In stages one and two, the emphasis was on micronutrients to help your body heal and reset. In stage three, you'll shift that focus and direct it toward honing your optimal macronutrient breakdown in terms of how many of your calories each day should come from fats, carbs, and proteins. In this stage, hands-on personalized coaching is truly advantageous. However, with some careful attention and notetaking, many of our clients can get close to their ideal balance. Being mindful is key here. With each new food you reintroduce, monitor and record how you feel emotionally and physically, in addition to any fluctuations in your weight. Some folks find they do better with higher amounts of fat in their diets; they are able to maintain their weight and feel great. While others, like Dan, tend to do better with higher carbs and lower fat in their daily intake.

Foods for Stage Three

In addition to the foods you ate in stage two, you can begin incorporating more into your diet. As you do, look for trigger foods—foods that cause a weight spike or some sort of physical discomfort. And introduce them slowly, just one or two new ones a day, so that it is easier to track how your body responds to each one.

Fruits (try increasing to three to four servings a day):

✓ Melons   ✓ Bananas

✓ Mango   ✓ Pineapple

✓ Grapes

Veggies:

✓ Peas   ✓ Pumpkin

✓ Carrots   ✓ Eggplant

✓ Squash

Proteins:

- ✓ Salmon
- ✓ Ahi Tuna
- ✓ Pork
- ✓ Lamb
- ✓ Moose
- ✓ Protein powders

Nuts and seeds:

- ✓ Almonds
- ✓ Cashews
- ✓ Nut butters and flours made from almonds, cashews, and coconuts
- ✓ Pistachio
- ✓ Walnuts

Other:

- ✓ Dairy (use extreme caution here; it is often inflammatory)
- ✓ Quinoa
- ✓ Dry wine
- ✓ Hard alcohol (remember: most mixers are loaded with sugar!)
- ✓ Olives
- ✓ Monk fruit
- ✓ Xylitol and erythritol as sweeteners in moderation

Weight Set Point Theory

An important part of stage three is the "lock-in." Now that you've lost a significant amount of weight (we guarantee at least twenty pounds during stage two, but most women lose between twenty-five and thirty, and men between thirty and forty), you will want to maintain it, which is what locking in helps do.

To lock in, you intentionally stay within two pounds of your new weight for three weeks while eating a significantly higher number of calories as you reintroduce the new foods. This strategy is often overlooked by weight loss programs, which is unfortunate because that might be why some people rebound and gain the weight they lost. Here's why: if you go on a plan with severe calorie restriction, after a while, your body starts to think you might be experiencing a famine, so your brain thinks, "If I'm only eating 500 calories a day, then I need to slow everything down and burn only 500 calories a day." Then, after you start eating more, your body stays in that 500-a-day burn rate as you eat more than 500 calories for a while, and that means you pack on more weight. So, after you lose a significant amount of weight the *re:vitalize* way, we suggest you give your body a break to let it stabilize at your low weight and high metabolic rate while you simultaneously eat significantly more energy. Essentially, this will trick the brain into thinking, "Oh, I can take in a normal number of calories each day AND stay twenty, thirty, or even forty pounds lighter." And *that* is what we want the body to do.

Three weeks is about how long it takes your body to adjust its metabolism and create a new set-point for where it thinks your weight should be. Failing to follow this stage exactly will put you at risk of failing to reset your metabolic rate properly.

If you are not at your ideal weight, you can repeat stages two and three until you do reach your goal.

We had a client come to us who had *already* lost and *kept off* over 100 pounds for more than ten years, which is really unheard of. As Dan spoke with him, he learned the man had used this very same approach. He'd punctuate thirty-to-sixty-day weight loss sprints with three to four weeks of maintenance, where he'd level off. This stair step approach is one of the most powerful ways to create *sustainable* weight loss, even if it feels counterintuitive to stop your progress for three weeks if you still have more weight to lose.

Stage Four

This is your new life! Here, you get to fear no food. Your metabolism will be fixed, so you can pretty much relax about eating. In this stage, you move from high support and less structure to full freedom and empowerment to enjoy the foods you love. The key is to continue your healthy lifestyle. To help with that, we encourage you to continue weighing yourself every day because sometimes we can slide back into old habits and let the weight creep back up on us. However, if you notice you have an upward change in your weight in this stage, you have the tools to reverse it: enter stage two for a couple of days to get back where you were.

Our most successful clients have discovered they can use elements from stages one through three in their weekly and monthly rhythms to help maintain their weight or continue to lose it should they overindulge too much on vacation or for some other reason. Here is one popular method many use to do that:

- Sunday through Wednesday: eat as if you're in stage two (intermittent fasting, limited protein, high veggies, limited fruit, no fats or oils)

- Thursday and Friday: eat as if you're in stage three (stage three foods, no intermittent fasting)

- Saturday: eat as if you're in stage one (enjoying fun foods like pizza or ice cream in moderation; other programs would call this a cheat day or cheat meal)

If trying to do something that structured seems more than you want to manage, make things easy on yourself. Try following the 80/20 rule: fuel your body well 80 percent of the time with foods that you enjoy and make you feel good, then for the remainder 20 percent, treat yourself in moderation. This is why *you don't have to fear food!* Once you make it through the first three stages, you have optimized your metabolism and addressed your body's biochemistry.

Now your body will want to maintain your new weight—as long as you don't overindulge *all* the time and *most* of the time (at least 80 percent) you do what we like to tell our clients to do: "fuel your body well." That means:

- If it came from a plant, eat it—if it was made in a plant, don't.

- Eat *food*, not food-*like* substances.

- Eat the rainbow—and we're not talking about Skittles! Have foods with a variety of color on your plate with each meal.

- The closer to nature, the better! Natural, as in nothing added or taken away.

- Stick to your foundational diet of vegetables and fruits

- Read *all* your labels.

In addition to weighing yourself every day, practice mindfulness. Being mindful about when, what, and where you are eating, and/or maintaining a journal or log where you record your diet and what's going on, will both be a tremendous advantage. They'll help you to tune into what's behind some of your nutrition choices—perhaps you'll see that certain negative emotions trigger cravings, or stress will encourage a slide, or maybe you'll discover at certain times of the day your body needs more fuel than others, or you may learn something else about yourself. Regardless, both mindfulness and journaling or logging will help you become aware of what is influencing you, and in doing so can support you to make healthier choices and strategies around eating.

No matter what though, one thing to always keep in mind is:

**A temporary return to old habits
does not mean failure!**

You can get back on the healthy wagon time and time again. It is always available to you. As Dan likes to say, "If you've quit, unquit." Just because you've stopped, doesn't mean you can't just restart. The most successful folks aren't perfect all the time, they are successful because they restart and get back into a rhythm quickly.

By the way, you can download our 7-Day Free Challenge e-book that rolls a lot of the elements of our program up into a one-week program folks can try at home. You can find it here: http://www. fearnofoodbook.com/.

YOU DON'T HAVE TO
DO THIS ALONE

Whether you are a local client who comes into one of our offices or you work with us remotely, one of the things we promise you is that you will not be alone on your weight loss journey. Our team will support you every step of the way.

We have recipes, shoulders to lean on, and the support structure you need to get you through this tough time, and we will celebrate with you when you win. As you'll see in the next chapter, having a little extra support can make a huge impact.

CHAPTER 9

BUDDY UP

 Marissa had been heavy for a number of years. This single mother worked out of her home, so not only was her job sedentary, but she didn't have many options for leaving and moving about.

She had tried numerous diets and programs—even HCG. As a former athlete, she knew what it takes to be physically fit. But she had a mental block that prevented her from connecting with what she really needed to improve her life in the long run. Or, to paraphrase what she said: she knew in her mind that she needed one thing, but in her heart, she needed ten cookies.

Still, she was on a spiritual journey and felt her faith was prompting her to take better care of her physical body. Then one day, she heard Dan when he was speaking on a TV show, when he said something that resonated with her: "people need to heal from the inside out." Without hesitation, she made the call to our clinic, began a program created for her, and lost sixty-four pounds.

She was elated, to put it mildly. As someone who looked at clothing from the aspect of "how much of me can I hide," she was surprised to find herself thinking differently about the way she dressed. She began to wear smaller clothes that flattered her and boosted her self-image even more. For the first time ever, she was comfortable using video cameras to talk to her clients. But one of the non-scale wins for her was to see how her daughter changed, too. Her little girl started wanting to snack on healthy vegetables with her mom.

Shining with new-found confidence, she impressed one of her clients so much that she was asked to do a presentation for a very large organization. In the past, she never would have done it—not without even thinking about whether her double chin was noticeable or if she looked chunky. But those wins were small compared to when her young daughter said she wanted to eat vegetables for a snack just like Mom!

From the sound of this story so far, you'd think Marissa was on top of the world. And she was, somewhat. One of the things that held her back was that she lacked support from her family. Her sister actually complained about her healthy food choices! And when she mentioned to her father how much weight she'd lost, he was unimpressed and told her she needed to lose more.

Fortunately, Marissa found a second family with the folks at our clinic. Marissa likened her weight loss to an inner battle, a war, where you need soldiers to back you up. She found our team at *re:vitalize* to be that army. The coaches were in trenches with her, and they were there to celebrate her wins.

WHAT DOES A WEIGHT LOSS COACH DO?

W e can't speak for every weight loss clinic, but at ours, our coaches wear several hats.

Cooking and Meal Preparation

We're pretty sure none of our clients have been five-star chefs (yet). Likewise, we know the last thing most people want to do is use every spare hour they have preparing foods. So we have numerous recipes, tips, and tricks our clients can follow.

Our coaches will make sure you get the ones that fit your personal profile and will even help you with creating meal plans so you never open the refrigerator door after a long day at work and wonder just what in the world you are going to make for dinner.

And if cooking isn't your thing, we do have meal-prep partners we can connect you with who are familiar with our methods and will create meals for you based on your profile.

Accountability

Once you are on your plan, having someone hold you accountable will be a huge help. Even our professional athletes enjoy and need accountability. We all do! So we'll ask you to text us each morning with your weight and other qualitative data. This allows us to make sure you're making meaningful weight loss progress daily.

And we do weekly check-ins, either in person or via teleconference. You'll get a biometric body composition and metabolic analysis during each of these check-ins so that our health coaches can assess your internal progress and make mid-course adjustments if necessary.

Problem Solving

It's not abnormal for someone trying to lose a lot of weight to hit a plateau where the scale just doesn't want to budge. Nor is it rare for someone to find it difficult at times to maneuver through their lives while still adhering to the requirements in stage two. For both situations, a coach is indispensable.

A good nutritional coach will be able to go over your trends and see where the plateau first began. Then they can help you figure out what you need to do to get the scale moving again. Frequently, that requires a "reset" day or two, where you eat only specific foods. Your coach will tell you what foods will work best for you and how long you should do the reset.

Plateauing

And as far as maneuvering through life—yes, our coaches know just how difficult stage two can be. In fact, all of them have been on the plan, not just to lose weight but to understand what our clients go through. So they are full of strategies and advice on how to handle large family events like out-of-town weddings or reunions. They know the impact getting the flu can have on you. They know what it's like to be exhausted from being up with the baby and all you want the next morning is a Danish with your coffee. So not only can they help you strategize your way through the situation, but their "been there done that" empathy will be an added source of strength to help you keep going.

MORE THAN LISTENING

A good nutritional coach isn't just interested in making sure a person loses weight. Our coaches build relationships with our clients by being present with them, listening to them, and creating trust between them, as well as holding our clients accountable for following through on the plan. And, when anyone should ever slip up and indulge when it isn't the best time to do so, our coaches don't scold or shame. They know we are all human; we need encouragement and kindness to continue on our paths.

One of the best ways a coach can help you on your weight loss journey is to encourage you to look at yourself with that same framework: with encouragement and kindness to yourself to continue on your path.

We thought it would be fun to include our Coaches' Convictions with you. Everyone on our team agrees to abide by these statements when they come on board with our organization.

OUR COACHES' CONVICTIONS AND CORE VALUES

These are our collective beliefs. We embody these in many ways, but they are also our aspirations—both who we are *and* who we're becoming.

Personal Connection

We build long-term, personal relationships by establishing trust through doing what we say we'll do, delighting clients through "wow" moments, encouraging them, problem solving with them, and celebrating their achievements.

The way we interact with our clients and each other speaks of our investment in relationships. We greet each teammate and client by name with a bright smile and acknowledging eye contact. Each client and teammate knows that "we are there for them." We are consistent in our processes, coaching, and the ways we treat others because consistency builds trust—and all lasting relationships have a firm foundation of trust.

Boldness for Good

We have a conviction that everyone is worth investing in—whether it's a client, teammate, or ourselves.

We dive in and risk helping others; we dig in to the uncomfortable conversations and situations to find lasting solutions. As Daniel Harkavay puts it in *Becoming a Coaching Leader*, "You don't need to have all the answers . . . but you do have to be willing to work through the situation, to follow up, to confront behaviors that do not line up with the stated convictions, and to encourage at all times."

We do not shy away from hard conversations. We have a responsibility to keep our clients and teammates accountable to themselves, their goals, and what they say they are going to do and achieve. We dig into clients' struggles as well as our own, being radically truthful yet equally graceful in the ways we encourage and coach.

We value both results *and* relationships, people *and* productivity. We risk having hard conversations for the good of others.

Eager Professionalism

Because we love our job and are passionate to help create positive change for our clients, we:

- dress professionally.

- do what we say we'll do by effective follow up, follow through, and follow back.

- smile, a lot.

- sound bright and professional and friendly.

- own solutions start to finish.

Passion for Positive Change

We are proud of our coaching staff—actually, we're proud of everyone on our staff. And not because they are good for the bottom line, but because they are truly caring, compassionate people who only want the best for every one of our clients.

From the moment someone walks in our door, they are sincerely made to feel welcomed and valued. Our staff goes the extra mile to build personal connections with everyone we work with. They know our program inside and out (most all of them have even gone through the program for themselves) and educate our clients on the why behind everything we do. They demonstrate a mastery of the routine, the foods, and the supplements, and educate our clients so well, they quickly become masters, too.

Our clients learn to come into our clinics and expect that level of compassion and education, and they always leave feeling supported and valued. That's just the way we do it and the way we feel a good coach should be.

We could go on and on for pages celebrating our staff, but what would be more helpful for you right now might be getting a taste of what our clients go through. So, up next, you'll find a handful of healthy recipes that are good for stage two of our plan.

CHAPTER 10

WHAT'S ON THE MENU?

If you're convinced you want to dabble a little bit in our methods, here are some recipes that work for many people in stage two of our plan. Vegetarian and vegan options follow.

VEGETABLE SOUP

INGREDIENTS

- 1 cup sliced celery
- 1 cup green beans
- 1 cup chunked zucchini
- ½ cup diced bell pepper
- 1 diced onion
- ½ cup spinach or collard greens
- ½ cup sliced mushrooms
- 8 cups water or chicken broth
- ¼ cup of Bragg's Amino Acids
- ½ tsp garlic powder
- 1 tsp thyme
- 1 tsp oregano

DIRECTIONS

Bring pot of water/broth to a boil.

Chop all vegetables and add to boiling water.

Add diced tomatoes and spices.

Cover and reduce heat. Let simmer until veggies are soft.

CHICKEN SALAD

This is one of Dan's all-time favorites. Great to eat with celery sticks!

INGREDIENTS

- 3–4 oz chicken breast
- 1 stalk of celery
- ¼ of an onion
- 3–5 radishes
- 1 cucumber
- 1 tsp yellow mustard
- 1 tsp Dijon mustard
- 3–4 tbs of coconut aminos
- Pink salt and pepper to taste

PREPARATION

Boil chicken breast in a pot of water.

As chicken boils, dice celery, onion, and radish in food processor.
Cut cucumber into slices.

DIRECTIONS

Shred boiled chicken with a fork or in the food processor.

Mix chicken, veggies, and condiments together in a large bowl.
Chill and serve with cucumber slices.

TURKEY SPINACH BOWL

INGREDIENTS

- 1 (10 oz) box frozen chopped spinach
- 3–4 oz ground turkey
- ¼ tsp minced garlic flakes
- ¼ tsp minced onion flakes
- Pinch of nutmeg and cayenne
- ½ tsp sage
- ¼ tsp fennel
- ¼ tsp thyme
- ⅛ tsp cinnamon
- 1 dropperful of SweetLeaf English toffee stevia

DIRECTIONS

Cook turkey in skillet until beginning to brown, then set aside.

Add water to skillet and bring to a boil.

Add spinach to skillet, then cover, reduce heat, and simmer for 10 minutes or until water is almost gone.

Stir in all spices, stevia, and turkey, and cook another 5 minutes.

BISON MUSHROOM MEATBALLS

INGREDIENTS

- 8 oz mushroom
- 3–4 oz bison
- 1 tsp liquid aminos
- 1 tsp lemon juice
- ¼ tsp ginger
- ¼ tsp curry powder
- ½ tsp onion powder
- Salt and pepper to taste

DIRECTIONS

Preheat oven to 400 degrees.

Line baking sheet with parchment paper.

Pulse mushrooms in food processor, then transfer to bowl.

Stir in lemon juice, liquid aminos, and spices.

Add beef to bowl and combine all ingredients together with hands.
Scoop mixture out by the spoonful into 8 mounds onto lined pan and
flatten into nugget shape.

Bake 20–25 minutes, or until cooked through.

TURKEY TOMATO SOUP

INGREDIENTS

- 2 cans diced tomato (14.5 oz)
- 20 oz ground turkey
- ½ cup organic chicken broth
- 1 white onion, chopped
- Sprinkle nutritional yeast flakes
- ½ tsp basil
- ½ tsp oregano
- ½ tsp garlic powder
- ½ tsp cayenne
- ½ tsp cumin
- Salt and pepper to taste

DIRECTIONS

In a large pot, bring the diced tomatoes and broth to a boil.
Add turkey and remaining ingredients to pot.

Cover and reduce to a low simmer.

Simmer for 25–35 minutes.

Serve in bowls and top with nutritional yeast.

BISON BOLOGNESE

INGREDIENTS

- 32 oz zucchini
- 20 oz ground bison
- 1 cup organic chicken broth
- 1 tbs minced onion
- Salt and pepper to taste
- ¼ tsp chili powder
- ½ tsp paprika
- ½ tsp cumin
- ½ tsp garlic powder
- ½ tsp basil
- ¼ tsp cayenne

DIRECTIONS

Wash and cut off zucchini ends. Slice onion.

Spiralize zucchini into noodles (or purchase pre-spiralized zucchini for quicker prep).

Sauté zucchini and onion in ½ cup of broth. Add ¼ tsp of spices. Brown bison in ½ cup of broth. Add remaining spices.

Serve zucchini noodles topped with bison in bowls. Salt and pepper to taste.

We actually had one couple (each lost over 60 lbs) who ate this meal almost every night with different protein because they loved it and could pile their plates as high as they wanted with delicious zucchini noodles and marinara.

BAKED LEMON FISH

INGREDIENTS

- ½ onion, thinly sliced
- 4–5 white fish or tilapia fillets
- ¼ tsp minced garlic flakes
- 1 lemon
- Pinch of cayenne
- 1 tbs Dijon mustard
- 1 tsp lemon juice
- Pink salt and pepper to taste
- Chopped parsley for garnish

DIRECTIONS

Preheat oven to 390 degrees.

Slice onions and lemon.

Wrap fish in foil with lemon, onions, garlic, and other seasonings.

Bake for 10–12 minutes, or until fish is just cooked. Remove from oven and transfer fish to serving plates. Garnish with parsley.

GRILLED FISH

INGREDIENTS

- 4 (4 ounce) tilapia fillets
- 3 cloves garlic, pressed
- 4 fresh basil leaves, chopped
- 1 cup white wine
- 1 large tomato, chopped
- Pink salt and pepper to taste

DIRECTIONS

Preheat a grill for medium-high heat.

Place the tilapia fillets on a large piece of aluminum foil.

Season with salt, pepper, garlic, basil, and tomato. Pour the wine over everything. Fold foil up around fish, and seal into a packet. Place packet on a cookie sheet for ease in transportation to and from the grill.

Place foil packet on the preheated grill, and cook for 15 minutes, or until fish flakes easily with a fork.

VEGAN
AND
VEGETARIAN
RECIPES

Many of our meat-eating clients have found the recipes below helpful to get more veggies into their diet. They simply add a protein serving to these dishes.

CHICKPEA SALAD

INGREDIENTS

- 1 can chickpeas, mashed
- Mustard (to taste)
- Nutritional yeast (to taste)
- Pink salt and pepper, other seasonings (to taste)
- Bell peppers, chopped

DIRECTIONS

Mix together and enjoy.

KALE AND BASIL PESTO

INGREDIENTS

- 1–2 cups kale, chopped
- 6–7 basil sprigs
- 2 cloves garlic
- ½ package of tofu, drained and pressed
- ½ cup lime juice or zest of lime.
- ¼ tsp pink salt
- Nutritional yeast (optional)
- Jalapeño (optional)
- ¼ cup water

DIRECTIONS

Mix all in blender or food processor and enjoy with veggies or on salad.

ROASTED BUFFALO CAULIFLOWER

INGREDIENTS

- Frank's Hot Sauce
- Head of cauliflower
- 1–2 beaten eggs for batter
- Nutritional yeast to coat cauliflower

DIRECTIONS

Preheat oven to 375 degrees.

Clean cauliflower and pat dry.

Break apart into florets.

Dip floret in the egg mixture first, then nutritional yeast to create "breading."

Roast for about 30 minutes or cook in an air fryer for 10 to 15 minutes.

Remove and toss in Frank's Hot Sauce, then cook another 5 minutes.

CHIA SEED PUDDING

INGREDIENTS

- ¼–½ tsp of chia seeds
- Enough water to soak chia seeds
- Stevia of your choosing (English toffee is one of our favorites)
- 1 cup fresh berries of your choosing.

DIRECTIONS

Mix all ingredients together in a bowl.

Refrigerate overnight.

ROASTED CHICKPEAS

INGREDIENTS

- 1 can chickpeas

Seasoning of your choice: pink salt, pepper, garlic powder, paprika, cumin, etc. (to taste)

DIRECTIONS

Preheat oven to 400 degrees.

Drain chickpeas and spread on a baking dish.

Sprinkle on seasonings.

Roast for 45 minutes, stirring every 15 minutes.

Top salads with these or eat by themselves as a snack.

CHICKPEA, QUINOA, OR BEAN CEVICHE

INGREDIENTS

- ½ cup drained chickpeas, cooked quinoa, or drained black beans
- 1 fresh-squeezed lime
- ¼ cup cilantro
- 1 medium tomato, diced
- 1 cucumber, diced
- ½ cup bell peppers, diced
- ¼ cup red onion, diced
- Fresh jalapeño or serrano—as much as you can bear!
- Pink salt and pepper

DIRECTIONS

Simple: mix all ingredients together!

LEBANESE LOUBIEH

Being Lebanese-American, this is one of Dr. Abood's favorites.

INGREDIENTS

- 5 cups green beans, trimmed and cut
- 1 large onion, peeled and finely chopped
- 3 large ripe tomatoes, finely chopped
- 4 tbs organic tomato passata
- 3 tbs mushroom broth
- 7 cloves garlic, whole and peeled
- 1 tsp pink salt

DIRECTIONS

In a large saucepan, add broth, garlic, and onion, and sauté over medium heat.

Add tomatoes and salt, continue to cook for 5 minutes.

Add tomato passata and green beans.

Cover, cook over low heat, and stir occasionally for 25 minutes.

CHEESE CRUSTED ASPARAGUS

INGREDIENTS

- 2 pounds fresh asparagus stalks, trimmed
- 1–2 tbs Simple Girl balsamic vinegar
- Juice of half a fresh-squeezed lemon
- ¼ tsp garlic powder
- Pink salt and black pepper to taste
- ½–¾ cup nutritional yeast

DIRECTIONS

Preheat oven to 425 degrees.

Take out a large sheet pan and line with parchment paper.
Lay asparagus stalks out on the pan evenly.

Drizzle balsamic vinegar and lemon juice over the asparagus, then evenly sprinkle garlic powder, salt, and pepper. Toss to coat.

Finish by sprinkling nutritional yeast over the asparagus. Again, toss until asparagus is evenly coated. The yeast should resemble a thin "crust" of cheese around each spear.

Bake in the oven for 12–15 minutes, depending on the thickness of the stalks.

Remove once crispy on the outside and enjoy!

TOFU SOUP

INGREDIENTS

- 1 pack of firm, organic tofu
- 1 cup sliced celery
- 1 cup chunked zucchini
- ½ cup diced bell pepper
- 2 cans diced tomato
- 1 cup green beans
- 1 diced onion
- ½ cup spinach or collard greens
- ½ cup sliced mushrooms
- 1 tsp yellow mustard
- 1 tsp Dijon mustard
- ¼ cup coconut aminos or Bragg's liquid aminos
- 8 cups water or mushroom broth
- Pink salt and pepper to taste

- ½ tsp garlic powder
- 1 tsp thyme
- 1 tsp oregano

DIRECTIONS

Bring broth to a boil. As it comes to temperature, dice any combination of veggies or add them to a food processor.

Add all vegetables to boiling broth.

Add diced tomatoes and spices.

Cover and reduce heat to simmer.

Cook until veggies are soft.

SPINACH AND BROCCOLI
ENCHILADAS

INGREDIENTS

- 10 oz chopped frozen spinach
- 1 onion, diced
- 12 oz broccoli, chopped
- ½ cup water
- 3 cups salsa (divided)
- 1 tsp garlic powder
- 1 tsp Simple Girl Southwest Seasoning
- 8 oz extra-firm tofu, drained and crumbled
  OR ground protein of choice (perhaps beef or bison)

- 2 tbs nutritional yeast flakes
- 8–10 cabbage leaves

DIRECTIONS

Preheat oven to 350 degrees. Thaw and drain the frozen spinach.

Over medium heat, sauté the onion, spinach, and broccoli in water until tender. Add 1 cup of salsa, garlic powder, and seasoning blend.

Remove from heat; stir tofu/protein and nutritional yeast.

Coat baking dish with ½ cup of salsa to prevent sticking.

Divide spinach and broccoli mix among cabbage leaves and spoon it down the center of each. Roll up the leaves and place seam-side down in the baking dish.

Spoon remaining salsa over top of the wraps.

Cover with foil and bake for 25 minutes, or until heated through.

CONCLUSION

Dan and I hope we've been able to shed some fresh insight on weight loss for you. It's not every day that you learn about the impact of stress on your weight and metabolism—nor is it often you hear that it's possible to reverse those effects to rev your metabolism back up to lose your excess weight.

But science aside, we hope one of the most important things you take away from this book is that your weight does not define who you are. It's just something that you need to deal with. And the faster you deal with it, the more quickly you will improve your quality of life. As I frequently say, "If you don't take care of your health, someone else will, and they usually have a scalpel in hand."

We also hope you realize you don't have to go it alone. In fact, it's not desirable for you to go it alone. Whether you call one of our clinics or find someone else, make sure you have the support structure you need. Having someone who has your back as you struggle to develop habits to eat foods you may not be accustomed to will be integral for you to stick to your plan, whatever it is you choose to do.

So set yourself up to succeed. Learn what makes a good plan, tap into your why, find motivation in knowing you are doing something to benefit not only yourself but the relationships you have with everyone in your life, and connect with someone to support and help you. You can do this!

APPENDIX A

POSITIVE AFFIRMATIONS

- I believe in myself.

- I appreciate that I want to change.

- I can change.

- I choose to change.

- I choose to be happy.

- I am the only one who gets to tell me how to feel and what to think.

- I value my opinion of me over the opinions of all others.

- I am only responsible for me and my thoughts.

- I have power over my thoughts.

- My goals are worthy of being achieved.

- I am worthy of achieving my goals.

- I love who I am becoming.

- My body is amazing.

- I accept my body in this way.

- I am eager to help my body become healthier and stronger.

- I release all fear, doubt, and judgmental thoughts.

- I choose to see the best in me.

- I choose to see the best in others.

- I believe in me.

- I am perfectly imperfect.

BEFORE AND AFTER ANALYSES

Actual Client Body Composition Biodata: Before and After Results

58 yo	6' 0"	Male			
	Before	After	Difference
Weight	232	192.4	-39.6
BMI Change/Improvement			-5.4
Body Fat % Lost			-9.1%
Visceral Fat Rating Improvement			-5.3
Cellular Hydration Improvement[1]			+4.9%
Metabolic Improvement[2]			-30 yrs

[1] Change in body water %
[2] As measured by metabolic age reversal/improvement

Actual Client Body Composition Biodata: Before and After Results

34 yo | 5' 8" | Female			
	Before	After	Difference
Weight	256.2	196.2	-60
BMI Change/Improvement			-9.1
Body Fat % Lost			-15.2%
Visceral Fat Rating Improvement			-7.2
Cellular Hydration Improvement[1]			+7.2%
Metabolic Improvement[2]			-40 yrs

[1] Change in body water %
[2] As measured by metabolic age reversal/improvement

Actual Client Body Composition Biodata: Before and After Results

29 yo | 5' 8" | Female			
	Before	After	Difference
Weight	262.2	238	-24.2
BMI Change/Improvement			-3.7
Body Fat % Lost			-3.3%
Visceral Fat Rating Improvement			-2.2
Cellular Hydration Improvement[1]			+2.1%

[1] Change in body water %

Actual Client Body Composition Biodata:
Before and After Results

46 yo I 5' 10" I Female			
	Before	After	Difference
Weight	263.4	230.4	-33
BMI Change/Improvement			-4.7
Body Fat % Lost			-4.3%
Visceral Fat Rating Improvement			-2.7
Cellular Hydration Improvement[1]			+2.6%
Metabolic Improvement[2]			-8 yrs

[1] Change in body water %
[2] As measured by metabolic age reversal/improvement

Actual Client Body Composition Biodata:
Before and After Results

52 yo I 5' 6" I Female			
	Before	After	Difference
Weight	181	144.6	-36.4
BMI Change/Improvement			-5.9
Body Fat % Lost			-10.6%
Visceral Fat Rating Improvement			-3.5
Cellular Hydration Improvement[1]			+6.5%
Metabolic Improvement[2]			-31 yrs

[1] Change in body water %
[2] As measured by metabolic age reversal/ improvement

Actual Client Body Composition Biodata: Before and After Results

	Before	After	Difference
Weight	290.8	256	-34.8
BMI Change/Improvement			-4.9
Body Fat % Lost			-9.7%
Visceral Fat Rating Improvement			-7.2
Cellular Hydration Improvement[1]			+4%
Metabolic Improvement[2]			-31 yrs

[1] Change in body water %
[2] As measured by metabolic age reversal/improvement

Actual Client Body Composition Biodata: Before and After Results

67 yo | 6' 0" | Male

	Before	After	Difference
Weight	264.6	211.8	-52.8
BMI Change/Improvement			-7.2
Body Fat % Lost			-5.8%
Visceral Fat Rating Improvement			-5.3
Cellular Hydration Improvement[1]			+2.4%
Metabolic Improvement[2]			-18 yrs

[1] Change in body water %
[2] As measured by metabolic age reversal/improvement

Actual Client Body Composition Biodata: Before and After Results

73 yo	5' 7"	Female			
	Before	**After**	**Difference**
Weight	183	150.4	-32.6
BMI Change/Improvement			-5
Body Fat % Lost			-5.4%
Visceral Fat Rating Improvement			-2.4
Cellular Hydration Improvement[1]			+2.9%
Metabolic Improvement[2]			-20 yrs

[1] Change in body water %
[2] As measured by metabolic age reversal/improvement

ACKNOWLEDGMENTS

This project would not have been possible without the many contributors, advisors, friends, and family that have supported both Dan and me through the process of bringing this work to life and the building and growing of our business. We've broken our acknowledgements up into a few sections: first, the folks both Dan *and* I want to thank together, then sections for folks I want to acknowledge specifically, and finally the people Dan wants to acknowledge.

FROM BOTH

Both Dan and I would like to foremostly thank our sincere and caring staff (past and present) who are the very heartbeat of the health revolution we're building, specifically: Becca Buster, Lauren Bastin, Alexis Pierce, Katie Lange, Janna Stevens, Tyler Herder, Tarah Stuart, Sansanee Perritt, Natasha Foster, Sheila Hrabchak,

Sam Abood, Ashley Hamman, Amy Blackwell, Stefanie Medley, Rachel Heronema, Jake Gorsky, Abbie Perizan, Ciara Erran, Linda Grisham, Pete Fischer, Celena Leland, Brandon Zenisek, Tracy Kopkas, Lindsay Bromfield, Kat Harrison, and Carrie Ailstock. You all embody and live our values so effortlessly, and we are truly honored to serve our clients alongside you.

Secondly, we want to thank all of you whom we're honored to count as clients, particularly those raving champions who continue to trust us with the health of their friends and family. Your consistent trust and referrals mean the world to us.

To those kind, generous individuals who contributed to this work specifically: Jenni Croft Badolato, Pete Rambo, Krista Coons, Bob Ree, Terry Xelowski, Steve Engram, Larissa Swartz, and Dr. Kari Anderson: thank you for your openness and candor in sharing your knowledge, struggles, successes, and transformation.

We are grateful for those who have used their platforms and massive spheres of influence to spread awareness of the life change happening through our weight loss programs. Particularly, Vince Marotta and Dan Bickley for starting the #BickleyandMarottaRevolution, and Paul "NeanderPaul" Munafo, Jenni Badolato, Tim Kempton, Eddie Johnson, Mike "Roc" Muraco, Shawn Crespin, Sarah Kezele, Double L, Miguel Montero, Dr. Jimmy and Bettina Chow, Jerod Cherry, Matt Fontana, and Greg Pruitt.

To our friends within professional athletics and the Phoenix Suns. To our friend, Dr. John Badalato: he was one of the first to welcome us to Phoenix. Dr. B has always been available to pick up the phone, talk, and introduce us to fellow physicians and playmakers across the valley. Thank you. To Aaron Nelson and Dr. Tom Fiel: thank you for trusting our program enough to share it with your colleagues, players, and patients. To Dan Costello and Doug Chisholm: thank you for being some of the most genuinely caring and authentic humans we've ever met, and thank you for being champions for us within the Suns and your network. Your friendship and partnership have meant so much to us, and we truly feel like part of the Phoenix Suns family.

A special thanks to Davis Jaspers for his marketing guidance and support as we opened up our second location.

This book would not have happened without our amazing publishing team. Specifically, we want to thank and acknowledge Lisa Shiroff: you made writing this book a true joy. Our sessions were lighthearted and full of laughs. You did such a wonderful job of capturing our thoughts and bringing them to life on paper. And to our entire team at Lioncrest/Scribe who helped bring this book to life. Particularly to Libby Allen, our Publishing Manager; Rachael Brandenburg, for an amazing book cover design; and Cristina Ricci, Brannan Sirratt, Kimberly Kessler, and the rest of the editorial and publishing team.

Thank you to our managers and reps at the various media outlets we've had the pleasure to partner with over the years. You've treated us with integrity and honesty, and continue to look out for our mutual best interests. Thank you to Kevin McElroy, Jasmin Duncan, Dawn Paugh, Kristen Leptich, Gabby Munoz, Tiffany Rickard, Trevor Emerson, the LSM digital team, and Sam Pines.

And to the many others who have helped us get here. Specifically to Jon and Bonnie Brovitz, for encouraging us to expand our thinking to see a grander vision for *re:vitalize weight loss* than maybe we saw ourselves; Rich Gale and Melissa Costello, for your wise counsel; Bob Goff, for challenging us to dream big and go for it; Simon Bromfield, for helping us design our first logo and brand identity in your spare time; and Dr. Barry Stahl, for coming to help in our clinics when we couldn't keep up with the demand.

FROM NOEL

I want to thank some of the people who have been with me over the years. Dr. Ray Wisniewski, who shared with me the concept of blending technology and weight loss. To Dr. Tom Insinna, who challenged me to think outside the box and live with integrity. A huge thanks to Tom and Ginny Baldini, who manage all aspects of my bookkeeping and accounting, allowing me to focus completely on my practice. To Lindsay Bromfield, who has been more than just an office manager—she is a friend; you anticipate my needs and work tirelessly to help.

FROM DAN

have more than a few people to thank. They say you are an average of the folks you spend your time with, and I give all credit for any modicum of success I've achieved to the great cadre of friends, family, and advisors I'm blessed to have by my side spurring me on.

To my wife, Danae: I truly could not have done any of this without you. Your friendship and love have been a staying force through all our crazy adventures together. You are always quick to remind me why we're doing hard things. Watching you lead and love our staff, make hard decisions, have crucial conversations, and work diligently to advance the common good have been one of the greatest joys of my life. You are an amazing woman, and I'm in awe of what you're able to accomplish with such grace, kindness, and love.

To my executive assistant, Robin Evans. You are so amazing at helping me stay free to focus on what's most important and keeping all the different balls in the air. We don't know what we'd do without you!

To my family: Mom, Dad, and Brian. Thank you for being such loyal fans of whatever crazy ideas and endeavors I've pursued (even if you didn't fully understand them). Whether it was my moving to Scotland to play rugby, lending me a few bucks to start that online beach clothing business, supporting us moving to a developing country only weeks after getting married—there has never been any doubt of your love and support.

There is one person who has been a true brother, business partner, partner in crime, and best friend from the start: Josh Bentley. You are the best salesperson I've ever met, and your optimism, enthusiasm, and belief always inspire me to be bold and go for it.

Of my teachers, mentors, and advisors there are many. Dr. Noel Abood (aka Doc, aka Noelly Choelly, aka El Gallo): thank you for giving me my shot and trusting us to partner with you and grow this practice. You've known me since I was just a knucklehead kid, and yet you still believed in me.

There are few men in my life as significant as Zach Clark. Thank you for investing in me, being so generous with your wisdom and guidance, for teaching me *how* to think about different things, and most importantly for your friendship.

Thank you to my friend Ryan Begelman for your coaching and being so quick with sharing your experience and helpful introductions. A special thanks goes to my first boss out of college, Cliff Croley, for teaching me the value of being resourceful with those four terrifying-yet-empowering words, "just figure it out." And to Elizabeth Heinz: your Godly counsel has helped me get out of my own way and out of my own head so I can be the best version of myself; thank you.

A few have helped me shift my paradigm around the role of business in culture. Thank you to Brent Warwick, Patrick Pace, and Curtis Powell for teaching me that organizations can be built, and business can be done in a way that is both profitable *and* people-focused that advance the common good.

And finally, to the many friends who are always quick with a kind and encouraging word, a distracting laugh, a needed brainstorm, a listening ear, or a helpful hand on this journey: Becca Buster, Lauren Bastin, Jeff Wright, Matt Simmonds, Chad and Krista Wallace, Ted Kruse, Darren West, Joe and Tina Atkinson, Mario Bundy, Jim Mullins and John Crawford, Jared Moore, and Dave Franco—thank you all!

ABOUT THE AUTHORS

Dr. Noel Abood, DC, is a weight loss and lower lumbar decompression pioneer with more than thirty years in the field. After surviving a heart attack at the age of forty-nine, Dr. Abood developed a wellness approach focused on personalized nutrition and metabolic health. He lost thirty pounds and gained a new perspective on sustainable health that became the premise for his weight-loss and wellness center, *re:vitalize.*

He maintained clinics in Ohio and Arizona, and is now based in Phoenix, where he has been chosen by the Phoenix Suns to be part of their nutrition team. Dr. Abood is an avid runner and cyclist, and he enjoys playing golf and tennis. He's been married for over thirty-five years and has two grown children.

Dan LeMoine is an entrepreneur and co-founder of *re:vitalize.* After earning a bachelor's degree in business management and two board certifications in nutrition, Dan and his wife, Danae, partnered with Dr. Abood to create the *re:vitalize* program.

Dan is a former competitive rugby player and now enjoys running marathons and cycling. He and Dr. Abood are both based in Phoenix, Arizona.

ABOUT *RE:VITALIZE WEIGHT LOSS*

Re:vitalize weight loss is revolutionizing how people lose weight and keep it off. Our customized approach to weight loss utilizes the latest biocommunication technology to remove the guesswork out of weight loss and fix the metabolism. The *re:vitalize* program uses their cutting-edge technology, compassionate expert coaching, and a comprehensive holistic foundation to give you a roadmap to long-term weight-loss success.

Find out more at: www.revitalizeweightloss.com.

ENDNOTES

1 https://www.cdc.gov/nchs/products/databriefs/db313.htm#:~:text=In%20 2013%E2%80%932016%2C%2049.1%25,%25)%20tried%20to%20lose%20weight

2 https://newsroom.ucla.edu/releases/Dieting-Does-Not-Work-UCLA- Researchers-7832

3 https://www.ncbi.nlm.nih.gov/pmc/articles/PMC5895712/

4 Frederich, Robert C., Andreas Hamann, Stephen Anderson, Bettina Löllmann, Bradford B. Lowell, Jeffery S. Flier. 1995. "Leptin Levels Reflect Body Lipid Content in Mice: Evidence for Diet-Induced Resistance to Leptin Action." *Nat Med* 1, no. 12 (December): 1311–4.

5 https://www.ewg.org/skindeep/

6 https://www.ewg.org/skindeep/ingredients/701514-COAL_TAR/

7 https://www.ewg.org/skindeep/ingredients/705335-PROPYLPARABEN/

8 https://www.ewg.org/skindeep/ingredients/702512-FRAGRANCE/

9 https://www.nih.gov/news-events/news-releases/brain-may-flush-out-toxins -during-sleep

10 https://womenshealth.obgyn.msu.edu/blog/fda-removes-hcg-weight-loss -products-market; https://www.fda.gov/consumers/consumer-updates/avoid -dangerous-hcg-diet-products

11 https://time.com/magazine/us/4793878/june-5th-2017-vol-189-no-21-u-s/

12 https://www.ncbi.nlm.nih.gov/pmc/articles/PMC2866597/

[13] https://www.healthline.com/health/depression/obesity-and-depression

[14] Lo Coco, Gianluca, Salvatore Gullo, Laura Salerno, and Rosalia Iacoponelli. 2011. "The Association Among Interpersonal Problems, Binge Behaviors, and Self-Esteem, in the Assessment of Obese Individuals." *Comprehensive Psychology* 52, no. 2 (March): 164–170.

[15] https://care.diabetesjournals.org/content/37/6/1544.full

[16] https://europepmc.org/article/PMC/3139753

[17] Keizer, Anouk, Monique A. M. Smeets, H. Chris Dijkerman, Siarhei A. Uzunbajakau, Annemarie van Elburg, Albert Postma. 2013. "Too Fat to Fit through the Door: First Evidence for Disturbed Body-Scaled Action in Anorexia Nervosa during Locomotion." *PLoS ONE* 8, no. 5 (May): https://doi.org/10.1371/journal.pone.0064602.

[18] Steele, Claude M. 1988. "The Psychology of Self-Affirmation: Sustaining the Integrity of the Self." Edited by Leonard Berkowitz. *Advances in Experimental Social Psychology* 21 (April): 261–302.

[19] Sherman, David A. K., Leif D. Nelson, and Claude M. Steele. 2000. "Do Messages about Health Risks Threaten the Self? Increasing the Acceptance of Threatening Health Messages via Self-Affirmation." *Personality and Social Psychology Bulletin* 26, no. 9 (November): 1046–1058.

[20] Cascio, Christopher, Matthew B. O'Donnell, Francis J. Tinney, Matthew D. Lieberman, Shelley E. Taylor, Victor J. Strecher, Emily B. Falk. 2015. "Self-Affirmation Activates Brain Systems Associated with Self-Related Processing and Reward and is Reinforced by Future Orientation." *Social Cognitive and Affective Neuroscience* 11, no. 4 (November): 621–629. https://www.ncbi.nlm.nih.gov/pmc/articles/PMC4343089/.

[21] Taber, Jennifer M., William M. P. Klein, Rebecca A. Ferrer, Erin E. Kent, and Peter R. Harris. 2016. "Optimism and Spontaneous Self-Affirmation are Associated with Lower Likelihood of Cognitive Impairment and Greater Positive Affect among Cancer Survivors." *Annals of Behavioral Medicine* 50, no. 2 (April): 198–209.

[22] https://www.nhs.uk/common-health-questions/lifestyle/what-are-the-health-benefits-of-losing-weight/

[23] Blackburn, George. 1995. "Effect of Degree of Weight Loss on Health Benefits." *Obesity Research* 3 (September): 211s–216s. Reference for 10%: NIH, NHLBI Obesity Education Initiative. Clinical Guidelines on the Identification, Evaluation,

and Treatment of Overweight and Obesity in Adults. Available online: http://www
.nhlbi.nih.gov/guidelines/obesity/ob_gdlns.pdf pdf icon

[24] https://medicine.wustl.edu/news/moderate-weight-loss-improves-heart-health/
#:~:text=A%20research%20program%20at%20Washington,but%20reverse
%20significant%20health%20problems.

[25] https://www.ncbi.nlm.nih.gov/pmc/articles/PMC2695566/

[26] Ang, Yee. 2018. "Reversibility of Diabetes Mellitus: Narrative Review of the
Evidence." *World Journal of Diabetes* 9 (July): 127–131.

[27] https://www.ncbi.nlm.nih.gov/pmc/articles/PMC3021364/

[28] https://academic.oup.com/jnci/article/112/9/929/5675519

[29] https://pubmed.ncbi.nlm.nih.gov/16983058/

[30] Faulconbridge, Lucy F., Thomas A. Wadden, Robert I. Berkowitz, David B.
Sarwer, Leslie G. Womble, Louise A. Hesson, Albert J. Stunkard, Anthony N.
Fabricatore. 2009. "Changes in Symptoms of Depression With Weight Loss:
Results of a Randomized Trial." *Obesity: A Research Journal* 17, no. 5 (February):
1009–1016.

[31] Kolotin, Ronette L., Martin Binks, Ross Crosby, Truls Østbye, James E.
Mitchell, Guilford G. Hartley. 2008. "Improvements in Sexual Quality of Life
After Moderate Weight Loss." *Int J Impot Res* 20, no. 5 (August): 487–492.

[32] https://www.cdc.gov/obesity/adult/defining.html

[33] https://consultqd.clevelandclinic.org/degree-of-obesity-relates-to-risk-of-post
-operative-complications-in-hip-and-knee-arthroplasty/

[34] https://www.cdc.gov/nchs/products/databriefs/db360.htm

[35] https://www.wsj.com/articles/weight-loss-is-harder-than-rocket-science
-11580396067

[36] Sievert, Katherine, Sultana M. Hussain, Matthew J. Page, Yuanyuan Wang,
Harrison J. Hughes, Mary Malek, Flavia M. Cicuttini. 2019. "Effect of Breakfast on
Weight and Energy Intake: Systematic Review and Meta-Analysis of Randomised
Controlled Trials." *BMJ* 364 (January). doi:10.1136/bmj.l42.

[37] https://www.healthline.com/nutrition/10-health-benefits-of-intermittent
-fasting#TOC_TITLE_HDR_4

[38] https://pubmed.ncbi.nlm.nih.gov/29700718/

[39] https://translational-medicine.biomedcentral.com/articles/10.1186/s12967-016-1044-0

[40] https://health-bath.co.uk/blog/four-ways-dehydration-inhibits-fat-loss-and-four-ways-to-fix-it/

[41] https://www.webmd.com/diet/sleep-and-weight-loss#1

[42] https://sparq.stanford.edu/solutions/use-smaller-plates-smaller-waist

[43] https://www.ncbi.nlm.nih.gov/pmc/articles/PMC4546438/

[44] Dr. Patrick Porter, "Reversing the Aging Process," recording, BrainTap Pro application, https://braintap.com/braintap-app/.

[45] Boyle, Marie. 2016. *Personal Nutrition*. 9th ed. Boston: Cengage Learning.

[46] https://www.ncbi.nlm.nih.gov/pmc/articles/PMC4488002/pdf/JNME2015-760689.pdf